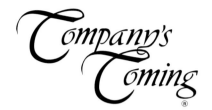

Superfoods Cookbook

Recipes for a Healthy Lifestyle

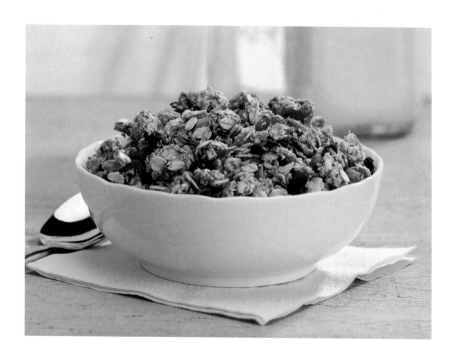

Jennifer Ogle • Patrick Owen
James Darcy • Jean Paré

Superfoods Cookbook

Copyright © Company's Coming Publishing Limited

First Printing June 2012

Library and Archives Canada Cataloguing in Publication

Superfoods cookbook / Jennifer Sayers ... [et al.].

(Healthy cooking series)

Includes index.

At head of title: Company's coming.

ISBN 978-1-897477-86-1

1. Cooking. 2. Health. 3. Cookbooks. I. Sayers, Jennifer

II. Series: Healthy cooking series

TX714.S346 2012   641.5'63   C2011-907660-8

Cover recipe: salmon with blueberry pan sauce, see page 133

Publisher's Note: The information contained within this book is not meant to replace professional medical advice and/or treatment.

Published by

Company's Coming Publishing Limited

2311 – 96 Street

Edmonton, Alberta, Canada T6N 1G3

Tel: 780-450-6223   Fax: 780-450-1857

www.companyscoming.com

Company's Coming is a registered trademark owned by Company's Coming Publishing Limited

We acknowledge the financial support of the Government of Canada through the Canada Book Fund for our publishing activities.

Printed in China

CONTENTS

INTRODUCTION

My Greens Are Better Than Yours

We all know instinctively what's healthy and what's not. Broccoli and salmon are healthy. Chips and fries: not so much. What's not so instinctive is knowing what foods are exceptionally healthy. National dietary guidelines of several countries invariably emphasize that we should consume more fruits and vegetables. In some of these food guides, we are told to favour some vegetables over others. In Canada's Food Guide, for example, we are told to include at least one dark and one orange vegetable in our diet each day. We are told specifically to "go for dark green vegetables such as broccoli, romaine lettuce and spinach," and "go for orange vegetables such as carrots, sweet potatoes and winter squash." The experts who came up with these recommendations used evidence-based science to determine which vegetables should figure predominantly in our diets. What does this mean for the colourless cauliflower or the purple eggplant we know are healthy? What makes the dark green and orange vegetables so special? The answer is that, calorie for calorie, dark green and orange vegetables are perhaps the most concentrated source of vitamins and minerals of any food. They are especially rich in vitamins A, C and K, calcium, potassium, iron and manganese.

Dark green and orange vegetables are also rich in phytochemicals, compounds that are not in the strict sense nutrients, but that are nonetheless absorbed and metabolized, and can influence our metabolism and physiology. Phytochemicals are usually expressed in plants as a defence mechanism against environmental stress, herbivory or infection. These same chemicals that help the plant survive through tough times also seem to help us ward off disease. Broccoli and kale, for example, contain potent anticancer phytochemicals called isothiocyanates that in the plant are used to repel herbivorous moths and other insects. Carrots and sweet potatoes are orange because of carotenoid pigments that play a vital role in photosynthesis. When we eat these compounds, they enhance our immune system, protect us from cancer and macular degeneration, and have potent antioxidant effects. These qualities are what differentiate a vegetable such as iceberg lettuce from a super vegetable such as spinach. Foods that offers more "bang for your buck" are what we like to call superfoods.

Would the Real Superfood Please Stand Up?

There is no official definition of what a superfood is, so the term is often used overzealously by manufacturers and aggressive marketing campaigns to sell a particular food product or supplement that has health benefits, oftentimes exaggerated to the status of a miracle food. Unsubstantiated health claims of products marketed as superfoods abound on the Internet and entice health-conscience but ill-informed consumers into paying big bucks for a product that sounds exotic or has a long ethnobotanical history but offers the same nutrients one might find in an apple. Many dieticians and nutritional scientists refrain from using the term "superfood" because they dispute the food's proclaimed nutritional and medical prowess. In legal terms, the term doesn't hold much water either, although its use has been regulated in some places. The European Union, for example, prohibited the use of the term "superfood" in 2007 unless it is backed up by evidence-based science and a specific medical claim. The term is nevertheless often used in popular media to describe nutrient-dense whole foods that many researchers, doctors and nutritionist believe can help prevent or treat diseases. The definition we are using in this book is "nutrient-dense whole foods that offer additional health benefits beyond simple nutrition."

We emphasize "whole foods" meaning foods that you would traditionally find in a garden or the produce aisle of your grocery store. Many well-known, inexpensive foods may easily be considered superfoods if research uncovers a health benefit. Phytochemical powerhouses like green tea and red wine have always been considered to have medicinal properties, so their pharmacological effects have naturally attracted attention from researchers. Tea and wine might easily have been the world's first superfoods. Other superfoods are recent additions that have been hyped by the media but are only supported by preliminary, yet very promising research. Açaí and goji berries are examples. They've been used traditionally for centuries by the Indigenous people of Brazil and the Himalayas, respectively, but they've only recently been introduced to the West. Like most berries, açaí and goji are

packed with nutrients and have exceptional antioxidant capacities, at least in laboratory tests, but they are not the miracle cure to all human diseases as some Internet sites claim. It'll take a few years for researchers to elucidate the berries' pharmacological properties in detail, but until then, they are included in the superfoods family based on their nutrient density, antioxidant capacity and anticipated health benefits.

Yet another group of superfoods are foods that we wouldn't necessarily think of as healthy at all. Chocolate is a perfect example. This sweet treat was always associated with sinful pleasure and, if we ate too much, guilt. As it turns out, research showed that the cacao nut contains an abundance of antioxidant polyphenols, many of which are also found in green tea. One cup of hot chocolate generates antioxidant activity that is five times greater than that of black tea, three times greater than that of green tea and twice as strong as a glass of red wine, and thus contributes to the prevention of cardiovascular disease and cancer. However, as soon as you add milk to the mix, most of these benefits disappear because of a change in polyphenol absorption. So dark chocolate with more than 70% cacao is considered a superfood, but milk chocolate with added sugar, is not.

The Family Goes to Pieces

Although we emphasize "whole foods" in this book, superfoods are characterized principally by their chemical composition; it isn't the single nutrient that counts, but the total effect of the food. A famous example is beta-carotene. When consumed from food sources, beta-carotene can be a potent antioxidant and provides us with vitamin A. When taken as a nutritional supplement however, beta-carotene may increase the risk of lung cancer in smokers. Researchers have possible explanations as to why a compound might behave differently in the body depending on its source, but the underlying message is clear: get your nutrients and phytochemicals from food.

The nutritional sciences are still in their infancy and there is still a lot we don't know about food. The effect of food is usually more, or quite different, from the sum of its parts. Foods have an extremely complex matrix of chemicals that interact with each other in ways that affect the way they are digested, absorbed, transported, metabolized, stored and excreted. Some compounds interact with our genes and can affect our metabolism, physiology and wellness. The field of nutrigenetics is a very young science that studies exactly these kinds of nutrient–gene interactions. The situation is further complicated if you add more than one food into the mix, which is almost always the case at mealtime. Cooking, baking, frying, steaming, grilling or any other processing method can further modify the composition and bioactivity of food compounds. There is much we need to learn about what we eat and how it affects us, but when it comes to health, take a hint from what we've been doing since the dawn of time: eat food.

We've evolved to eat food, not nutrients. Our digestive system is a master at breaking down protein into its constituent amino acids, polysaccharides into their constituent sugars, and fats into diacyglycerides and fatty acids. We have transporters and carriers for every vitamin and mineral along different sections of our digestive system. As we digest, food breaks down to release nutrients gradually so that we can absorb them efficiently. Compare this to how a multivitamin might be absorbed. Copper absorption is enhanced by the ingestion of animal protein but is inhibited by high levels of zinc and cadmium. Low levels of copper will in turn inhibit iron absorption,

which is enhanced by vitamin C. Excess vitamin C is excreted because it is water-soluble and can't be stored. This interplay between nutrients and our bodies may seem complex to us, but to our digestive system, it's child's play.

Superfood Family Ties

Everyone knows someone who is a "one-upper"—a person who insists that whatever you've done or experienced, they've done or experienced it better than you have. The one-uppers in the superfoods family are called "functional foods." A rapidly growing segment of the food industry is aiming to make it easier for consumers to boost their health and prevent chronic disease by fortifying products with nutrients that promise benefits. This means that grocery shopping will get a lot more complicated. If green tea is a superfood, then green tea ginger ale would be a functional food. Would one derive the same benefits from drinking fortified soda that they would from tea? Food manufacturers will try to make you believe so, but regulatory bodies carefully monitor exactly what is allowed to be said on health claim labels. To date, Canada only allows six health claims, which tend to be general and vague. For example, products that have added calcium and vitamin D can carry a label linking those nutrients to a decreased risk of osteoporosis. But the health claim becomes a little dubious if the product is a juice, vitamin water or granola bar that contains high amounts of sugar. In the U.S., labelling laws are a lot less strict, and you may find an entire line of orange juice with splashy labels claiming that it reduces cholesterol, boosts your immunity or nourishes your brain. As appealing as these goods may sound, you should be aware that companies seldom put enough nutrients in a product to make any difference to a person's health. In the end, the choice is yours. Functional foods may supply extra nutrients, but the food as a whole must be evaluated for its overall nutrition and health qualities.

Forest for the Trees

Superfoods are usually natural foods that are low in calories, minimally processed and free from any additives, hormones, pesticides or antibiotics. However, although they are exceptionally healthy foods, they are not everything. What to include in your diet is almost as important as to what to exclude. You won't feel much different if you down a handful of blueberries after polishing off a plate of fries. The same goes for other lifestyle factors such as stress, sleep and exercise, all of which are tightly linked with diet. In today's world, hardly anybody gets enough sleep. Chronic sleep deprivation has profound effects on hormones that control metabolism, appetite, mood, concentration, memory retention and food cravings. It is associated with high blood pressure, elevated stress hormone levels, irregular heartbeat and compromised immune function, and it drastically increases your risk of obesity and heart disease. Poor sleep increases levels of cortisol, a stress hormone that has several beneficial effects on the body, but when chronically elevated, becomes extremely problematic. Cortisol promotes the storage of fat around the abdominal area, decreases libido and decreases the production of serotonin. Eating sugar and starches causes an increase in serotonin levels, which explains why several people eat sweets when stressed or staying up late. Because serotonin enhances calmness, improves mood and lessens depression, this sets up cravings for additional carbohydrates and sweets.

Health is a web. A diet loaded with superfoods is an extremely important strand, but it won't mean much to your well-being if there is an imbalance in your sleeping patterns or stress levels. Address any deficiencies you may have in your life that may impede your path to optimal health so that you may reap all the benefits superfoods have to offer. No part can be ignored.

In a Super-nutshell

The information in this book gives you ammunition against cardiovascular disease, obesity, type 2 diabetes, frailty and a host of other complications that come with poor health. But information is one thing; implementation is another. The recipes in this book provide delicious examples of how superfoods can be incorporated into your diet. They are easy-to-follow, simple and made from ingredients that you'll be able to find at your local grocery store. With these foods, you'll get all your essential vitamins and minerals, and you'll be exposed to a barrage of healthy phytochemicals that will help you ward off disease. The health benefits of the superfoods listed in this book are evidence-based and free from exaggerated claims. For some foods, a solid body of research exists based on human clinical trials. For others, research has just begun, but preliminary findings strongly suggest that the foods are useful in health maintenance and disease prevention.

As more and more is known about the foods we eat, no doubt the list of superfoods will grow. The diversity of superfoods included here allows you to experience a variety of different cuisines and flavours, and perhaps introduce a few foods you've never tried before. Get cooking as soon as possible and keep on cooking. Consistency in good habits is the key to health and the sooner you start, the sooner you'll feel better. We hope that this book inspires you to be the best that you can be and to become the healthiest you've ever been in your life.

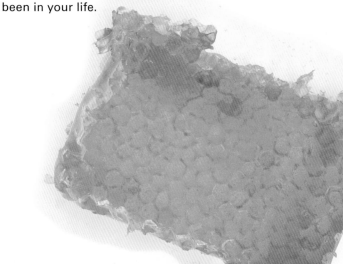

THE UNORDINARY BERRY

The Original Superfood

It would be impossible to have a book about superfoods and not start off with berries. An overwhelming body of research has now firmly established that eating these small, soft-bodied fruits has a positive and profound impact on human health, performance and disease. Berries, which are commercially cultivated and commonly consumed in fresh and processed forms, include blueberries, blackberries, black and red raspberries, cranberries and strawberries. Lesser known but important in the traditional diets of North American indigenous peoples are chokecherry, highbush cranberry, serviceberry, silver buffaloberry, arctic bramble, bilberries, black currants, boysenberries, cloudberries, crowberries, elderberries, gooseberries, lingonberries, loganberries, marionberries, Rowan berries and sea buckthorn. Recently, the popularity of exotic berries such as the Himalayan goji berry, Brazilian açaí berry and the Chilean maquie berry has increased dramatically.

The consumption of berries has a positive effect on a variety of diseases, including heart and cardiovascular disease, neurodegenerative and other disease of aging, obesity and certain cancers such as esophageal and gastrointestinal. Although berries are packed with vitamins, minerals, folate and fibre, their biological activities are largely attributed to their high levels of phenolic phytochemicals. These include flavonoids (anthocyanins, flavonols and flavanols), tannins (condensed tannins such as proanthocyanidins, and hydrolyzable tannins such as ellagitannins and gallotannins), stilbenoids and other phenolic acids. For example, cranberries have a unique proanthocyanidin structure that prevents bacteria from adhering to cell walls, which explains their effectiveness in the treatment of urinary tract infections.

Overjoyed about Flavonoids

Berries are considered nutrition powerhouses primarily because of their flavonoid content. These powerful antioxidants scavenge harmful free radicals and reduce inflammation. Berries rank higher than any other fruit or vegetable according to the ORAC (oxygen-radical absorbing capacity) test, and among them, açaí is at the top. The ORAC value is a method of measuring and comparing the antioxidant capacity of different foods and supplements. In theory, foods with a higher ORAC value are more effective in neutralizing free radicals and reducing degenerative disease, but the exact relationship between the ORAC value and its health benefits has not been established. In any case, research has established that blood concentrations of flavonoids and other phenolic acids are much too low to have a noticeable antioxidant effect. Instead, flavonoids are extensively metabolized and are further converted by the gut flora into related compounds that persist in the blood and accumulate in specific parts of the body. It is often these metabolites that have a biological effect, often other than as antioxidants. They can reduce inflammation, regulate the activities of metabolizing enzymes, repair DNA damage and even modulate gene expression. As a result, flavonoids can affect the pathways and processes that lead to cancer development. In addition, some berry flavonoids can sensitize tumour cells to chemotherapeutic drugs and provide protection from toxic side effects. As far as anticancer food goes, nothing beats berries.

Flavonoids may also oppose the action of enzymes called secretases that are involved in the destruction of nerve cells and may be elevated in neurodegenerative disease. So if you need to remember where you left your car keys, first remember to eat your bowl of berries.

Among the best-studied flavonoids are the anthocyanins, pigments that give berries their attractive yellow, orange, red and blue colours. Particularly abundant in dark berries such as blueberries and açaí, anthocyanins have potent antioxidant activity, anti-inflammatory activity and the ability to inhibit the oxidation of low-density lipoproteins, a key step in reducing the risk of cardiovascular disease. When it comes to this superfood, the darker the berry, the more potent its power.

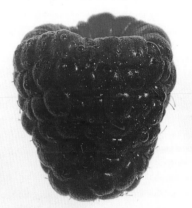

Love is a Berryfield
Berries can be eaten fresh, canned or frozen. Look for colourful, firm, ripe berries with no sign of mold or rot. Frozen berries retain all the nutritional qualities of fresh fruits, but they lose their firmness once they thaw.

It is clear from the wealth of research done to date that berries are potent agents in disease prevention and health maintenance. Many exotic or traditional wild berries still need to be evaluated scientifically, but advances in research techniques will allow us a better understanding of the mechanisms of how they affect our biology. One thing is certain—if berries are not a regular item in your diet, you need to start including them. They'll definitely add colour to your plate, and to your life.

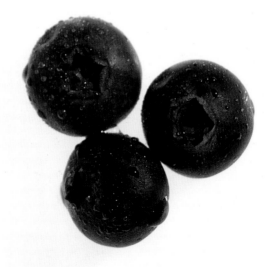

Açaí Berry

From the rainforests of the Amazon comes a berry that has been used for centuries to make a dark purple beverage, often referred to locally as "poor-man's juice." Açaí reached the North American market in the mid-2000s amid a flurry of claims that its juice was helpful for weight loss, detoxification, health promotion and disease prevention. Much of the increase in popularity stems from the development of several new products in the U.S. that are flooding the market for natural health products. Ironically, the "poor-man's juice" has become the rich man's high-dollar marketing campaign. Açaí does indeed have the highest superoxide free radical scavenging ability yet found for any food plant according to the ORAC Assay, although its hydroxyl radical scavenging activity was relatively poor. The concentration of antioxidants in açaí is roughly 10 times that of red grapes, and the berry contains 10 to 30 times more anthocyanins than red wine. Despite this, açaí does not seem to outperform other antioxidant-rich berries in regard to its biological activities. Some initial studies have shown that açaí is able to destroy leukemia cells in a cultured dish, but no studies have been done to substantiate its claim for weight loss. As far as we know, no novel compound has been found in açaí, but that doesn't take away from the fact that it is a highly nutritious, antioxidant-rich superfood that has the same potential health benefits as other berries, albeit with a higher price tag.

Brazilian Açaí Bowl with Granola

Serves 2

14 oz (398 mL) frozen açaí pulp

2 large bananas, *divided*

½ cup (125 mL) soy or almond milk

¼ cup (60 mL) raw honey (or agave nectar)

½ cup (125 mL) Good-for-You Granola (see p. 108)

Let açaí sit at room temperature for about 10 minutes to soften slightly. Coarsely chop 1½ bananas. Combine açaí, chopped banana, soy milk and honey in a blender. Purée until smooth (it should be quite thick). Divide among 2 deep bowls. Thinly slice remaining banana. Top açaí with banana slices and granola.

Honey contains at least 181 known substances that bestow it with strong antioxidant abilities. When it comes to a honey's antioxidant power, the darker the better. The quality of the honey depends on the flowers visited by the bee because the honey retains their fragrance and other properties. Buckwheat honey, one of the darkest, full-bodied varieties, has more than 20 times the antioxidant activity of sage honey, one of the lightest-coloured honeys. For the most health benefits, choose raw honey over pasteurized; the pasteurization process destroys many phytonutrients and enzymes.

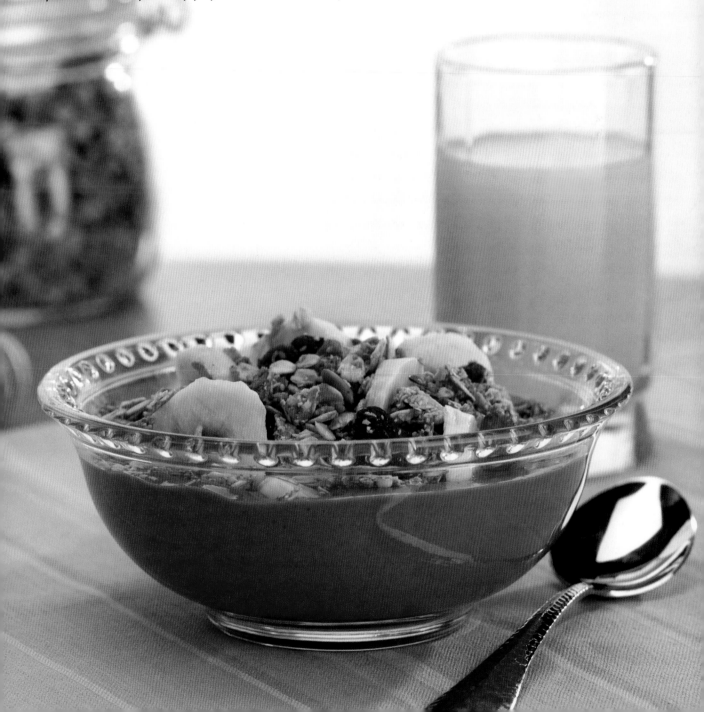

Rainforest Smoothie

Serves 2

7 oz (200 g) açaí purée or juice (frozen or thawed)

1 mango, chopped

1 cup (250 mL) chopped papaya

1 cup (250 mL) coconut water (see Tip) or papaya juice

Combine all ingredients in a blender. Purée until smooth. Divide among 2 glasses.

Tip

To get the coconut water out of a coconut, cut the husk off the bottom to expose the harder shell. You'll see 3 eyes. Punch holes in 2 of these with a sharp object like a screwdriver or corkscrew (one will be soft enough to poke through easily, the other one will be harder). Turn upside down and drain the water from the coconuts through a sieve (or drain, then strain) to get any bits of shell out.

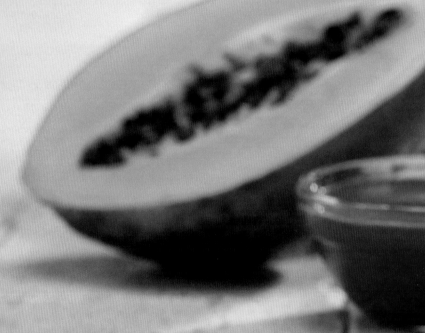

The açaí berry takes its name from Iaçí, the daughter of an Incan tribe leader who, after declaring that newborns must be sacrificed to offset a severe food shortage, learned of Iaçí's pregnancy. The child was born and sacrificed, and a devastated Iaçí locked herself in her hut without food or water. One night, the tribe leader heard his daughter's cries from the forest and ran to find her dead by a slender palm tree. She had a smile on her face, and her eyes were open, gazing upwards. Above, the tribe saw a bountiful cluster of dark purple fruits, which would become the diet of the tribe and save them, and their newborns, from starvation.

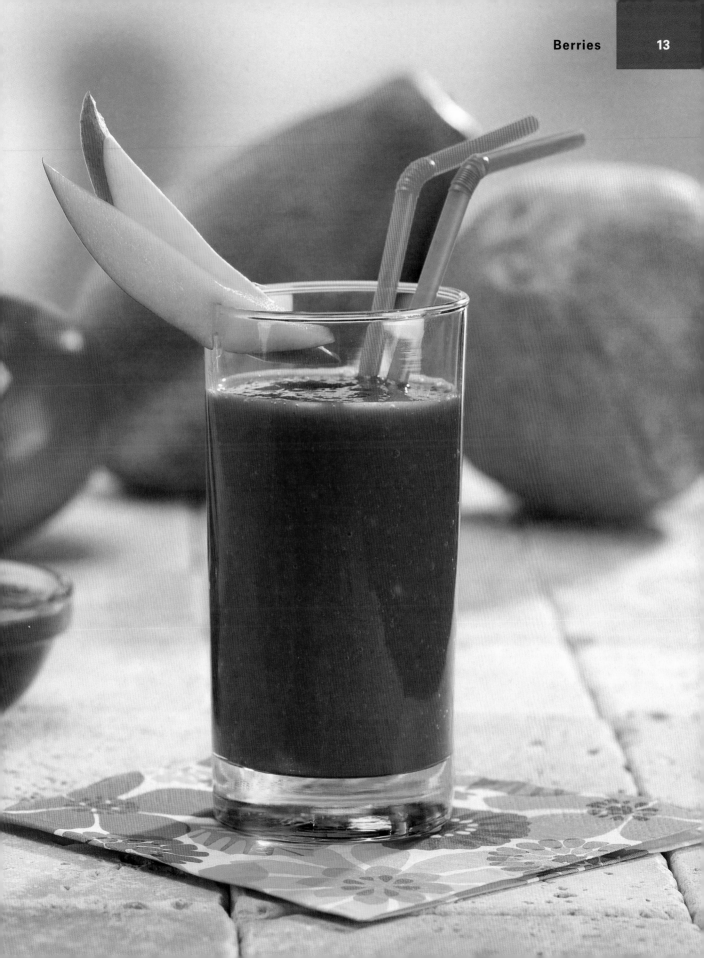

Blueberries

Britain's Royal Air Force pilots reportedly ate blueberries during World War II because the berries improved their night vision and allowed them to complete their missions with greater accuracy. Whether this story is true or not, it prompted European scientists to research the effects of blueberries on night vision. Numerous studies have since shown that blueberries improve nighttime visual acuity, increase adjustment to darkness and may even be beneficial against macular degeneration. The macula is an area in the centre of the retina that contains specialized cells responsible for seeing colour and fine detail. Past the age of 65, one in four people develop macular degeneration, which is caused by oxidative damage to the macula. The anthocyanins in blueberries not only prevent free radical damage by virtue of their antioxidant activity, but they also strengthen the blood vessels behind our eyes. Blueberry consumption is also associated with improved memory, learning and general cognitive function, including reasoning skills, decision-making, verbal comprehension and numerical ability. Emerging research also suggests that blueberries may help slow the decline in mental faculties that is often seen in aging and might even provide protection against disorders such as Alzheimer's and Parkinson's.

Blueberry Salsa

Makes about 3 cups (750 mL)

1 Tbsp (15 mL) lime juice

½ tsp (2 mL) salt

¼ cup (60 mL) cilantro

2 tsp (10 mL) minced hot chili pepper

2 cups (500 mL) blueberries

½ cup (125 mL) diced jicama, cut into ¼ in (5 mm) pieces

2 green onions, thinly sliced

Combine lime juice and salt in a medium bowl. Stir until salt has dissolved. Add cilantro and chili pepper. Stir to combine. Add blueberries, jicama and green onion and toss to combine. Serve as a side dish or as a topping for savoury grilled dishes, such as fish, as shown in the photo.

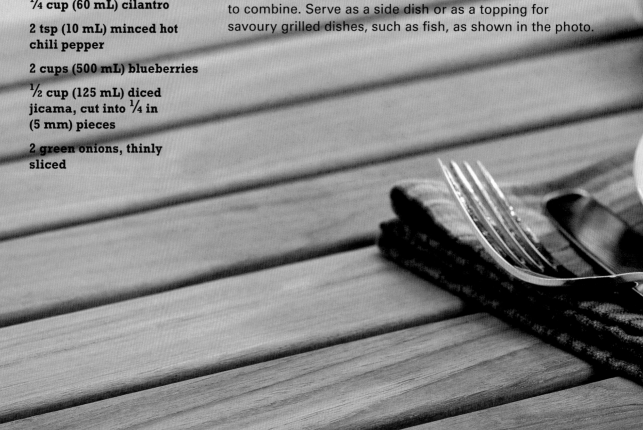

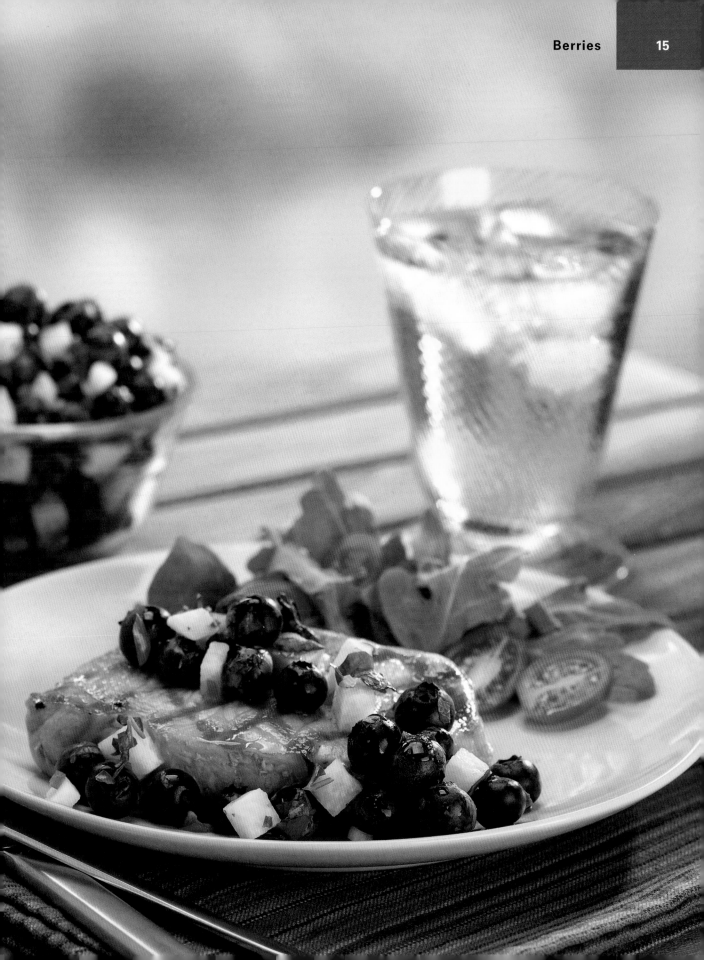

Spinach and Berry Salad with Honey Mustard Vinaigrette

Serves 4

1½ tsp (7 mL) unseasoned rice vinegar

1 Tbsp (15 mL) raw honey

1 tsp (5 mL) Dijon mustard

sea salt and pepper

3 cups (750 mL) baby spinach leaves

½ head of radicchio, torn into bite-size pieces

½ cup (125 mL) blueberries

½ cup (125 mL) sliced strawberries

½ small red onion, thinly sliced

2 Tbsp (30 mL) sunflower seeds

Combine vinegar, honey and mustard in a small bowl. Whisk well. Add salt and pepper to taste.

Combine spinach, radicchio, blueberries, strawberries and onion in a large bowl. Drizzle with dressing and toss to coat. Sprinkle sunflower seeds over top and serve immediately.

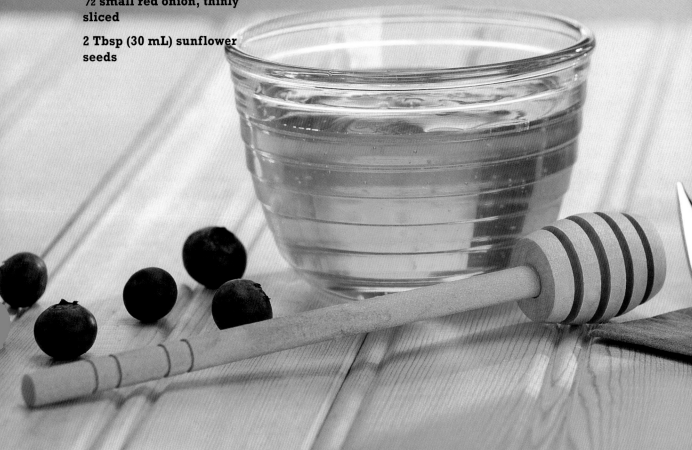

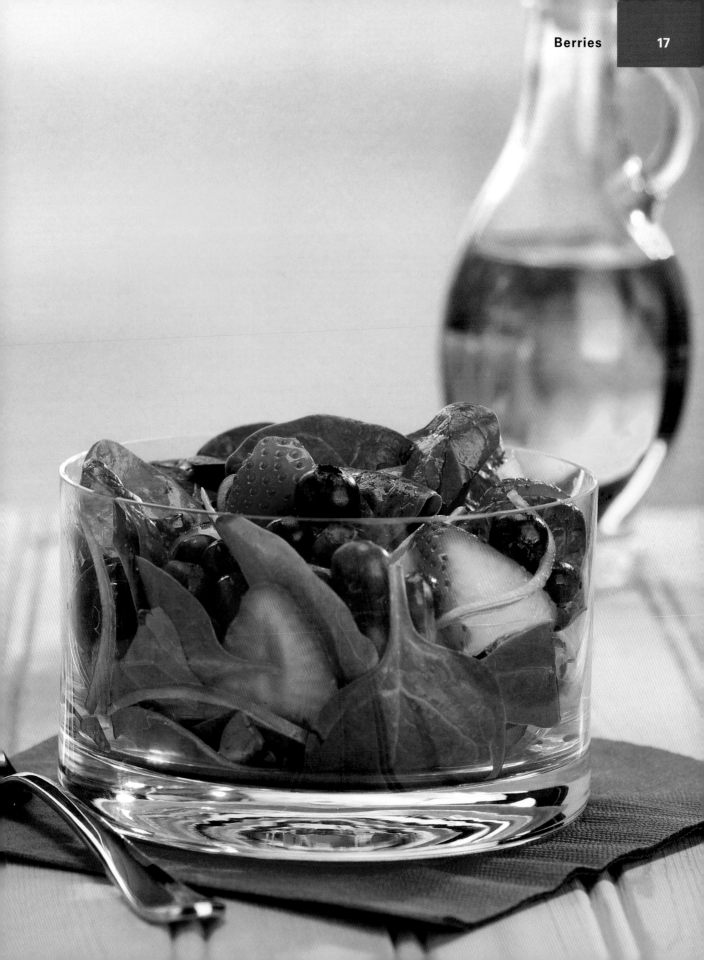

Cranberries

Native to North America, cranberries are perhaps best known as an accompaniment for the Thanksgiving turkey, but traditionally they were used extensively by indigenous peoples both as a food source and medicinally in poultices to heal wounds and stop bleeding. Current research indicates that cranberries have anti-inflammatory properties, especially in relation to the stomach, digestive tract and gums, and they are high in antioxidants, which combat cell-damaging free radicals. The berries also contain proanthocyanidins that inhibit bacteria from sticking to the stomach lining, preventing urinary tract infections and possibly stomach ulcers. Similarly, the proanthocyanidins may prevent bacteria from sticking to teeth, reducing the production of plaque and therefore protecting against peridontal diseases. Most of the nutritional and health benefits of cranberries are found in the whole, fresh (or frozen) berry, not in the juice or the dried version; to really take advantage of what cranberries have to offer, choose fresh!

Quick Fruit Compote

Makes 3 cups (750 mL)

¾ cup (175 mL) white grape juice

½ cup (125 mL) coarsely chopped dried apricot

1 large pear, peeled and cut into ½ in (12 mm) pieces

1 medium apple, such as McIntosh, peeled and diced

1 medium orange, peeled and cut into ½ in (12 mm) pieces

1 cup (250 mL) fresh or frozen cranberries

1 Tbsp (15 mL) orange juice

Combine grape juice, apricot, pear and apple in a medium saucepan. Bring to a boil. Reduce heat to medium-low and simmer, uncovered, for about 5 minutes, until softened. Add orange and cranberries. Stir gently, and cook for about 5 minutes until cranberries begin to split. Stir in orange juice.

Tip

If necessary, add up to another ¼ cup (60 mL) of white grape juice to get the consistency you want.

Tip

This versatile compote can be served hot or cold, as a dessert or as a condiment. It makes a great topping for pancakes or yogurt.

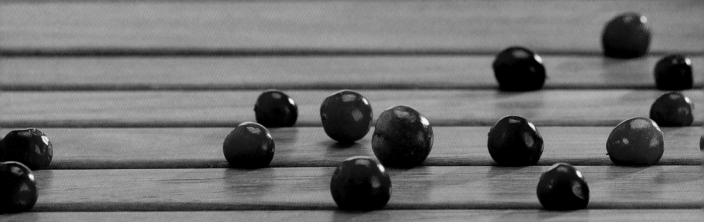

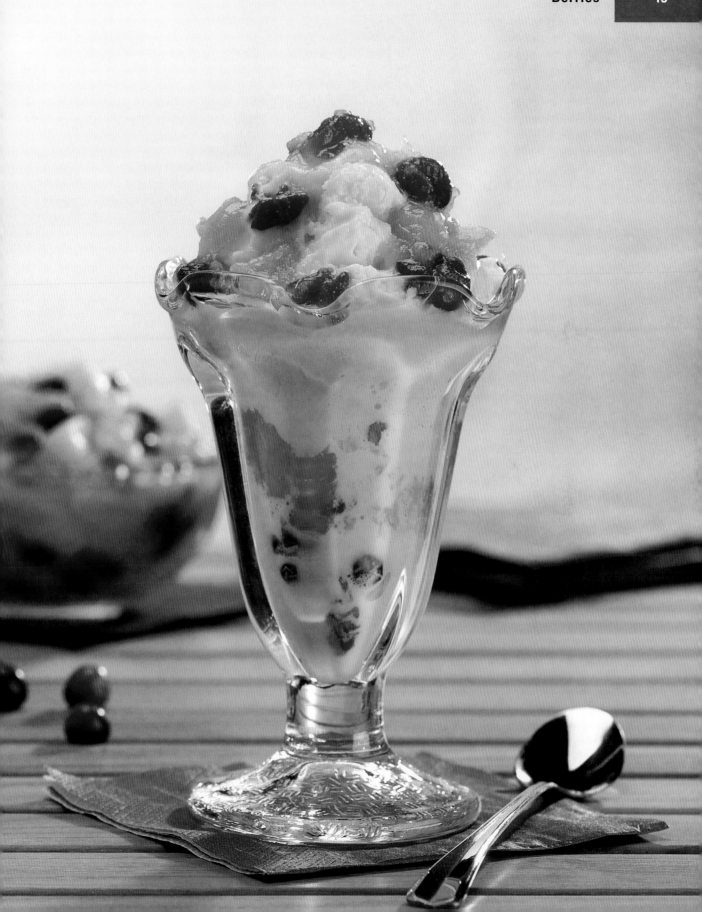

Cranberry Apple Cabbage

Makes 5 cups (1.25 L)

6 cups (1.5 L) shredded
cabbage, lightly packed

1 cup (250 mL) chopped
fresh (or frozen, thawed)
cranberries

1 diced, peeled apple, such
as Granny Smith

1 cup (250 mL) thinly sliced
red onion

2 bay leaves

$\frac{2}{3}$ cup (150 mL) apple juice

$\frac{1}{4}$ cup (60 mL) maple syrup

2 Tbsp (30 mL) apple cider
vinegar

1 Tbsp (15 mL) canola oil

$\frac{1}{4}$ tsp (1 mL) salt and
pepper

Combine cabbage, cranberries, apple, onion and bay leaves in a $3\frac{1}{2}$ to 4 quart (3.5 to 4 L) slow cooker. Combine apple juice, syrup, vinegar, oil, salt and pepper in a medium bowl. Add to slow cooker and stir. Cook, covered, on Low for 5 to 6 hours or on High for $2\frac{1}{2}$ to 3 hours. Remove and discard bay leaves. Serve as a side dish.

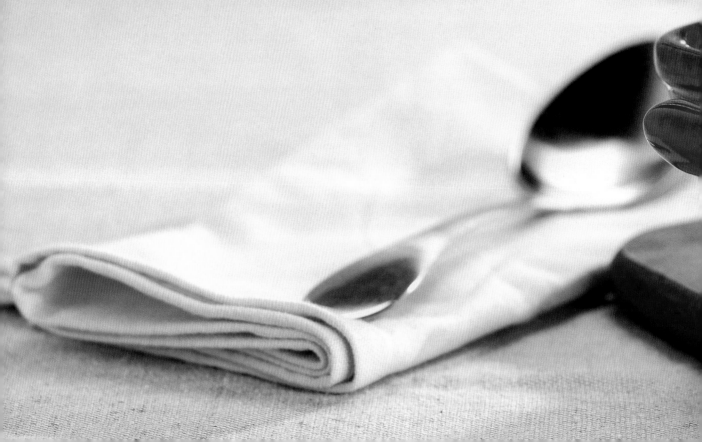

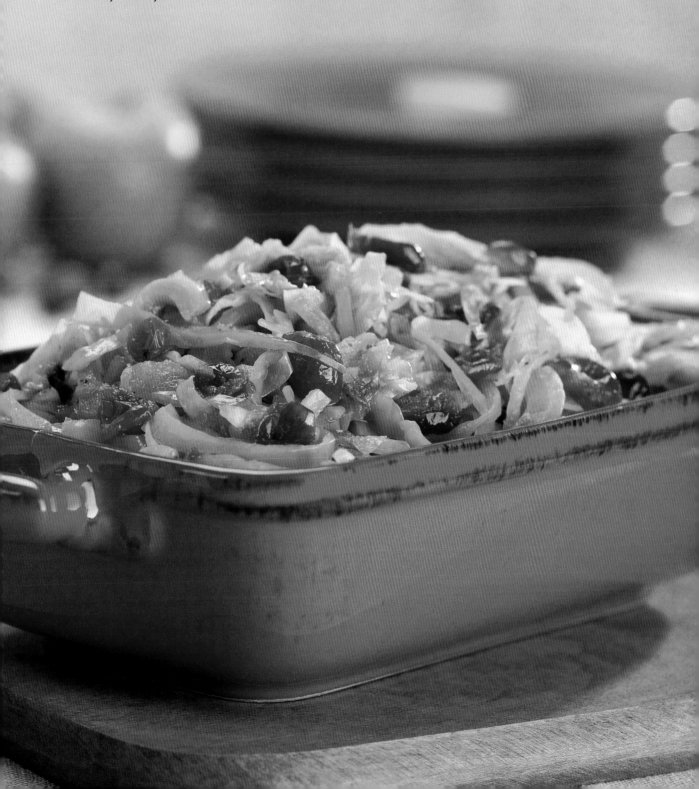

Although cranberries were never recorded as being part of the first thanksgiving, they are often associated with this holiday and symbolize the Earth's abundance.

Goji Berries

From the Himalayas comes the goji berry, which belongs to the nightshade family, so it is high in the carotenoids lutein, zeaxanthin and lycopene. These pigmented compounds are important in eye health and allow the eye to adapt more rapidly to darkness, a property that, along with resident antioxidants, may have therapeutic value in vision-related disease such as macular degeneration and glaucoma. Like açaí, goji has been marketed in the West as a potent superfood with several unsubstantiated health claims, especially attributed to its polysaccharide content. Beyond the hype though, it is nevertheless a highly nutritious berry with a long history of culinary use in China. The dried berry is usually cooked before consumption and is added to meals, soups, teas and tonics. Make sure to buy goji products that are organic, as some controversy exists about the overuse of pesticides and fungicides used in goji cultivation.

Goji Berry and Coconut Sauce

Makes about 2 cups (500 mL)

½ cup (125 mL) goji berries

½ cup (125 mL) coconut water (see Tip)

½ lemongrass stalk

1 cup (250 mL) young coconut meat

2 tsp (10 mL) finely grated ginger

2 Tbsp (30 mL) chopped fresh basil

2 Tbsp (30 mL) chopped fresh cilantro

pinch of sea salt

black pepper to taste

Place goji berries in a small bowl. Add coconut water. Set aside to hydrate for 1 hour.

Smash lemongrass stalk against a cutting board with flat side of a knife, then slice thinly crosswise. Transfer goji berries and soaking liquid, lemongrass, coconut meat and ginger to a blender. Purée until smooth. If using at room temperature or chilled, stir in basil, cilantro, salt and pepper to taste. If warming, add salt and pepper to taste, but stir in herbs just before serving. Store, covered, in refrigerator for up to 3 days. Serve chilled or at room temperature to dress salads or as a dip for veggies, or warmed over grilled or steamed fish or veggies.

Tip

In a pinch, substitute 1 cup (250 mL) organic coconut milk for the coconut water and coconut meat, and soak the goji berries in the coconut milk. The flavour will be slightly different but delicious nonetheless.

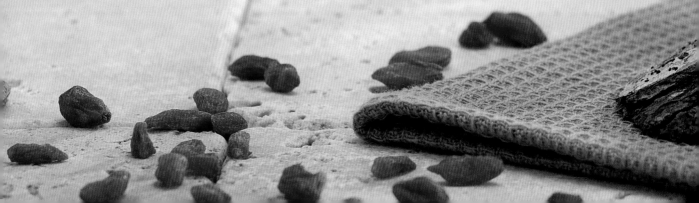

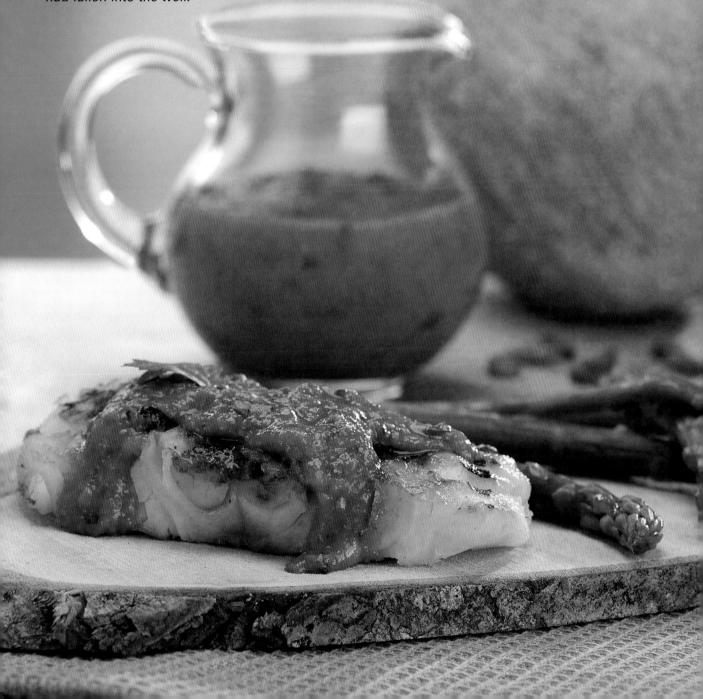

Tibetan folklore claims that ingesting too many Goji berries causes too much laughter, and a handful in the morning will make you happy all day. According to legend, the berry was discovered by a scientist who was studying an ancient society living in the remote regions of the Himalayas. He attributed their unnaturally long lives and health to prolonged ingestion of water spiked with goji berries that had fallen into the well.

Gingered Goji Berry Jam

Makes about ¹/₂ cup (125 mL)

¹/₂ cup (125 mL) goji berries

1 tsp (5 mL) finely grated lemon zest

1 tsp (5 mL) finely grated ginger

2 tsp (10 mL) agave nectar

Place goji berries in a small bowl. Add water to cover. Set aside to hydrate for about 30 minutes. Drain and reserve soaking water. Combine goji berries, lemon zest, ginger and agave in a blender. Purée until smooth, adding a little soaking water if necessary to get the blender going. Store, covered, in refrigerator for up to 1 week.

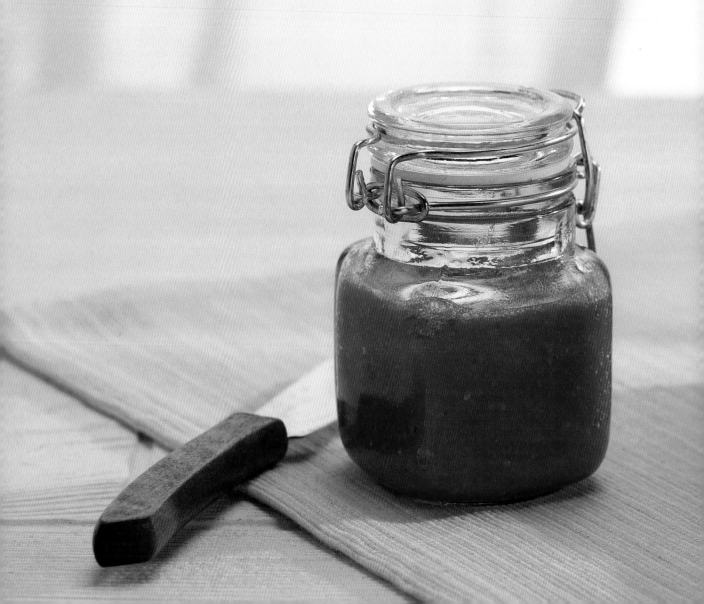

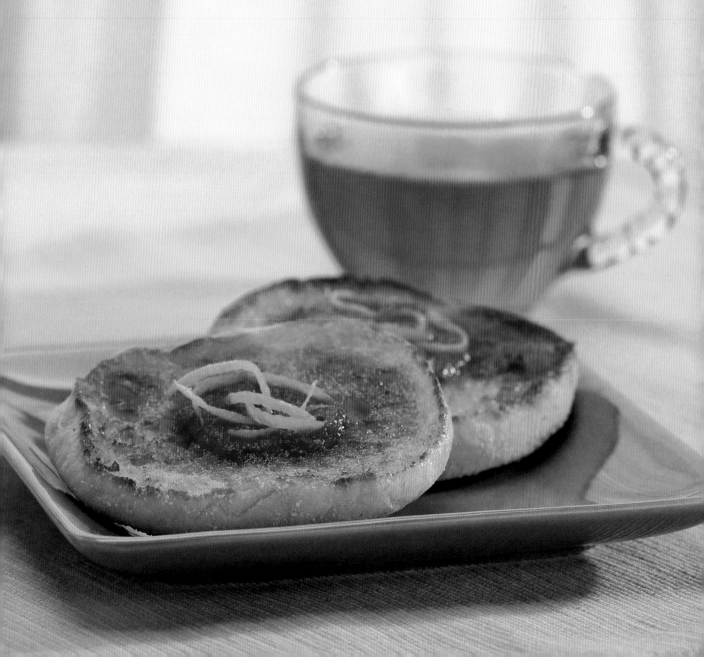

Agave nectar, also called agave syrup, is made from the sap of several species of agave plant, including blue agave (Agave tequilana), *the same species that gives us tequila. It is used as a sweetener and can be a healthier alternative to sugar or other highly processed sweeteners like corn syrup. Agave nectar is sweeter than sugar and can have more calories, depending on the manufacturer, but because it is so sweet, a little goes a long way. It is made primarily of a type of fructose called inulin, which does not cause the spike in blood sugar levels that is seen with sugar.*

Raspberries and Blackberries

Members of the *Rubus* genus, raspberries and blackberries grow on shrubs with prickly canes. The fruits are not true berries—they are aggregate fruits meaning that each "berry" is actually a bunch of drupelets held together by fine hairs. Raspberries, and to a lesser extent blackberries, contain ellagic acid, which can prevent the growth of tumours and induce apoptosis. It may also help the liver remove some carcinogens from the blood and protect against birth defects. Both types of berries contain anthocyanins, antioxidants that improve brain function and protect against macular degeneration, and both are excellent sources of vitamin E, which helps protect the heart and arteries. Raspberries are high in pectin, a type of fibre that helps control blood cholesterol levels, and unlike many other fruits, they do not cause spikes in blood sugar.

Mixed Berry Smoothie

Serves 2

½ cup (125 mL) goji berries

1 cup (250 mL) orange juice

½ cup (125 mL) blackberries

½ cup (125 mL) raspberries

½ cup (125 mL) blueberries

½ cup (125 mL) strawberries

1 apple, chopped

2 tsp (10 mL) bee pollen, *divided*

Place goji berries in a small bowl. Add orange juice and set aside to hydrate for about 1 hour.

Transfer mixture to a blender. Add berries and apple. Purée until smooth. Divide among 2 glasses. Sprinkle each glass with 1 tsp (5 mL) bee pollen.

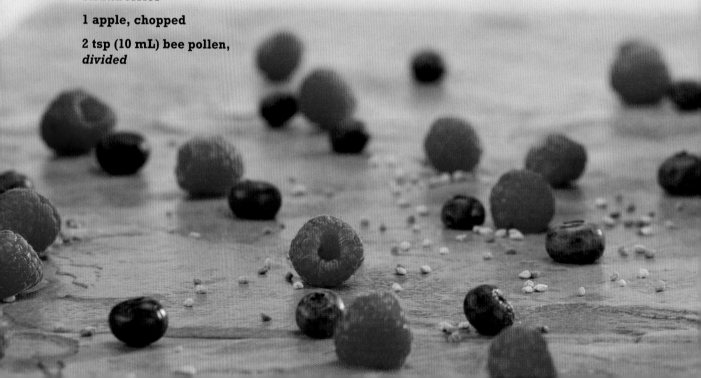

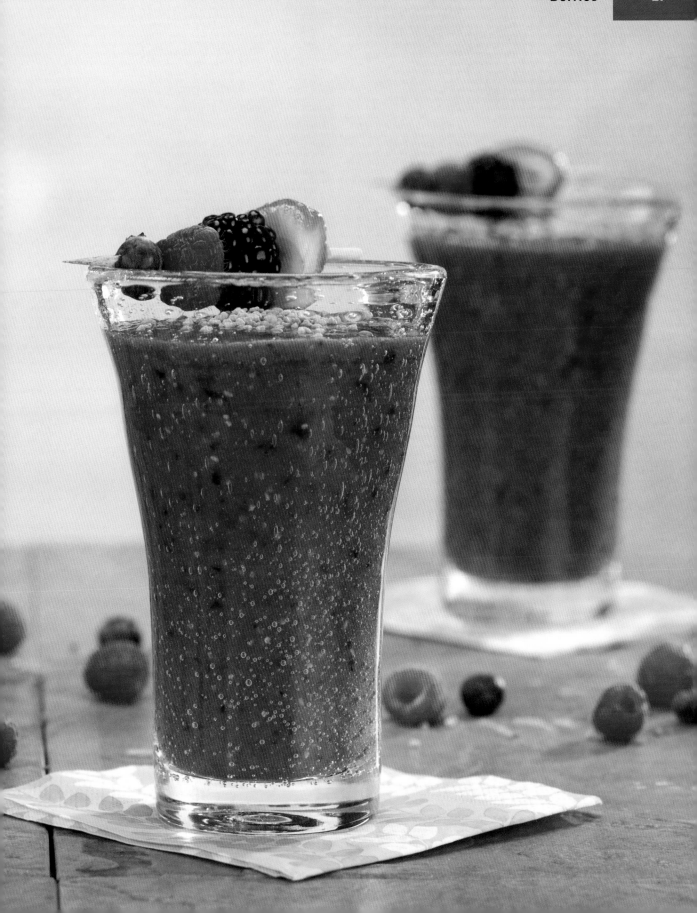

Raspberry and Spinach Salad

Serves 4

1¼ cup (300 mL) raspberries, *divided*

2 Tbsp (30 mL) raspberry (or red wine) vinegar

1 Tbsp (15 mL) olive oil

1 Tbsp (15 mL) honey

1 tsp (5 mL) Dijon mustard

¼ tsp (1 mL) pepper

5 cups (1.25 L) baby spinach leaves

1 cup (250 mL) thinly sliced button mushrooms

⅓ cup (75 mL) sliced almonds, toasted

Combine ¼ cup (60 mL) of raspberries, vinegar, oil, honey, mustard and pepper in a blender or food processor until smooth.

Combine spinach, 1 cup (250 mL) raspberries, mushrooms and almonds in a large bowl. Drizzle with dressing and toss gently to coat.

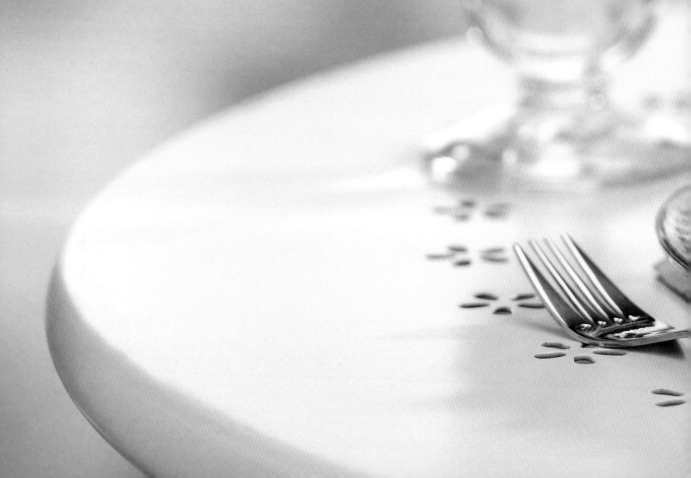

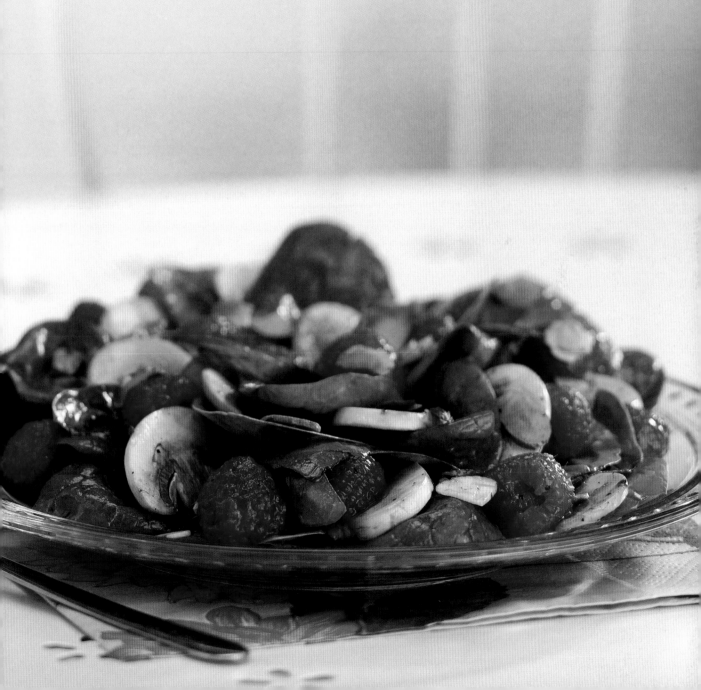

Raspberries, according to Greek legend, were discovered while the Olympian gods were searching for berries on Mount Ida, thus the Latin name Rubus idaeus. In Christian art, the red juice represented blood, which because it runs through the heart, symbolized kindness. Native Americans also associated the juice with blood and often used raspberries in medicines associated with childbirth and pregnancy.

GRAPEFRUIT THE GREAT FRUIT

The Forbidden Fruit

If it hadn't been for Captain Shaddock, a 17th-century English ship commander, grapefruit (*Citrus* x *paradisi*) may never have made its debut as a superfood. In 1693, Shaddock brought the ancestor of the grapefruit, the pomelo (*C. maxima*), from Malaysia and Indonesia to the West Indies. The fruit was bred for the first time in the New World in Jamaica, but the grapefruit that we know today most likely originated as a natural hybrid between the pomelo and the Jamaican sweet orange (*C. sinensis*). Welshman Reverend Griffith Hughes came upon the hybrid in Barbados in 1750 as he was searching for the mythical tree of good and evil of the Garden of Eden; when he saw the hybrid, he thought he had found the tree he was seeking, and he named the fist-sized bright yellow fruits "the forbidden fruit." The name stuck for a while in the region, where the fruit was also called "the shaddock" or "shattuck," after the good captain. The common English name "grapefruit" first appeared in 1814 when botanist John Lunan remarked that the fruit grew in clusters similar to grapes.

The New Kid on the Block

The grapefruit is arguably the youngest fruit in the superfood family. Barely 300 years old, the fruit didn't make an appearance in North America until 1823 when it was brought to Safety Harbor, Florida, from the Bahamas by Count Odette Phillipe. New grapefruit varieties, including those with pink and red flesh, were developed in the early 1900s. The fruit's popularity took some time to grow. The American gardening encyclopedia originally referred to it as "think-skinned and worthless." The U.S. stock market crash of 1929 and the ensuing Depression were the catalyst that introduced grapefruit to the wider public. When the welfare board handed out free grapefruits to those with orange food stamps, families who encountered the fruit for the first time had no clue how to eat it. The board received frequent complaints from people who had cooked the fruit for several hours and still found it too tough to eat. From then on, however, the grapefruit slowly and more frequently appeared as a breakfast favourite. Still considered new and exotic, the grapefruit also became a popular cocktail at dinners. Retrieving the juicy wedges, though, often caused the most inconvenient splashes on shirts and bosoms, and, inevitably, in the eyes. This problem was quickly resolved with the invention of the grapefruit spoon and the grapefruit knife,

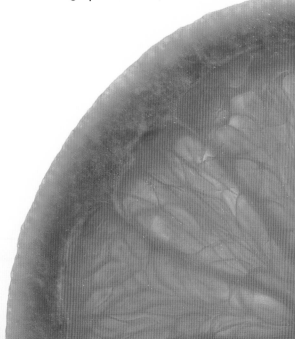

independently invented by clever grapefruit lovers who likely received a few too many painful wayward squirts in the eye. By the 1950s and '60s, most households owned a set of grapefruit spoons. Other eye-saving contrivances that never took off included the umbrella spoon and the squirt guard, both of which appeared in the *Modern Mechanix* magazine in the 1930s.

Mean Medicine

With only 66 to 84 calories per serving, grapefruits are loaded with vitamin C, calcium, potassium and magnesium, and the membranes are a good source of pectin, a soluble fibre helpful in reducing LDL cholesterol and improving insulin resistance. Pink and red grapefruits are particularly rich in pro-vitamin A and lycopene, a powerful antioxidant that has been extensively studied for its anticancer properties. Grapefruit seed extract is sold in health food stores as an antifungal remedy, and an infusion of the grapefruit flowers is used as a treatment for insomnia. The fruit contains high levels of spermidine, a simple polyamine necessary for cellular growth and maturation. As we get older, levels of spermidine drop, and animal studies strongly suggest that consumption of this compound significantly prolongs lifespan. When it was fed to mice in their diet, biological markers of aging decreased significantly, and when spermidine was added to cultured human immune cells, they also lived longer. Had Reverend Hughes known this, he might have called grapefruit "the fruit of the tree of life" instead of the foreboding "forbidden fruit."

MEDICAL WARNING: Grapefruit is known to interact with a number of prescribed medications, often increasing their effective potency. The flavanone naringin increases a drug's bioavailability by inhibiting the intestinal enzyme CYP3A4, basically causing a medication overdose. The drug interactions became known in 1989 when a group of Canadian researchers studying a blood pressure drug were shocked to discover that drinking a glass of grapefruit juice dangerously increased the drug's potency. Grapefruit interacts with many widely used drugs, often with no serious consequences, but in some cases it can be fatal. Common cholesterol-lowering medications such as Liptor, Mevacor and Zocor interact with grapefruit and can lead to the serious and sometimes fatal muscle disorder rhabdomyolysis. Grapefruit juice can also interfere with the metabolism of selective serotonin reuptake inhibitors (SSRIs), such as Prozac, used to treat depression. If you're taking multiple medications, you should be particularly careful and consider avoiding grapefruit juice altogether. Consult your pharmacist to find out whether grapefruit juice interacts with any of your prescribed medications.

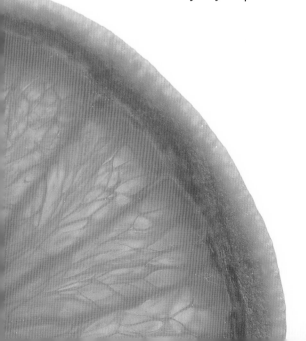

Ginger Honey Grapefruit

Serves 4

4 oz (115 g) ginger, peeled and finely grated (see Tip)

¼ cup (60 mL) raw honey

2 red grapefruit

2 tsp (10 mL) bee pollen, *divided*

Place grated ginger between 2 layers of cheesecloth. Working over a small bowl, squeeze firmly to extract juice. Discard ginger pulp. Add honey to ginger juice, and whisk to combine. Ginger honey can be kept covered in refrigerator for up to 2 weeks; stir before using.

Cut grapefruit in half. Run a sharp knife between flesh and pith of each half, being careful not to cut through skin. Cut between membranes and flesh to separate each section, but leave them in place. Transfer grapefruit halves to 4 plates. Drizzle 2 tsp (10 mL) of ginger honey over each half and sprinkle with ½ tsp (2 mL) bee pollen.

Tip

A microplane-style grater works best for grating ginger, but if you don't have one, coarsely chop the ginger then purée it in a food processor or blender.

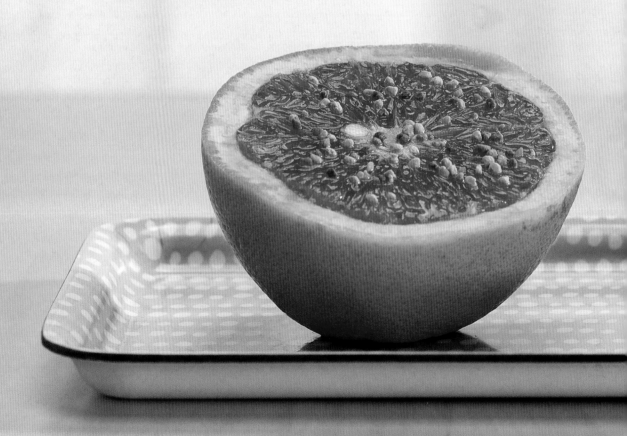

The Diet Craze of the Good Ol' Days

The Grapefruit Diet has been around since at least the 1930s but it wasn't until the '70s that it became a diet craze. Also called the Hollywood Diet or the Mayo Diet (though it was not associated with the Mayo Clinic), the diet was a short-term, quick-weight-loss plan based on the premise that compounds in the grapefruit interacted with protein and triggered fat loss. Actress Angie Dickinson, when asked in 1985 what kept her so young, responded: "So far I've always kept my diet secret but now I might as well tell everyone what it is. Lots of grapefruit throughout the day and plenty of virile young men at night." Virile young men aside, it is possible that there is some truth to the grapefruit's weight loss claim. In a small 2006 study, researchers found that the addition of a half grapefruit or 4 oz (115 mL) of juice with meals resulted in an average weight loss of 3 lbs (1.4 kg) in 12 weeks, with some participants losing 10 lbs (4.5 kg). The study was funded by the Florida Department of Citrus, however, so the reliability of the results is questionable. Otherwise, there is no solid scientific basis to the claim that grapefruit has special fat-burning enzymes or weight-loss attributes.

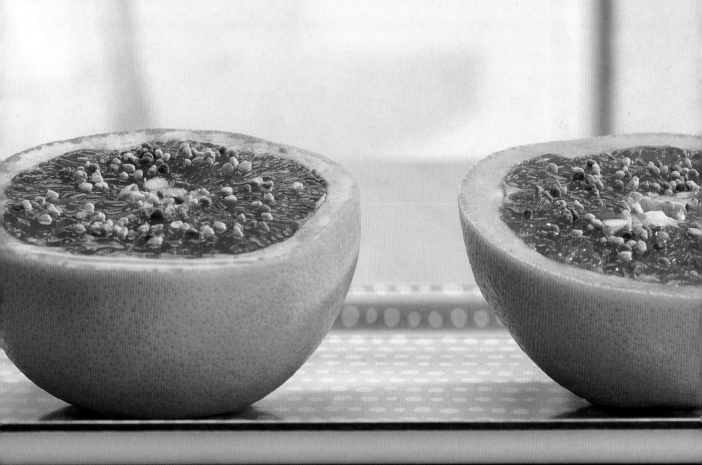

Thai-style Grapefruit Salad

Serves 4 to 6

1 tsp (5 mL) canola oil

3 shallots, very thinly sliced

1 Tbsp (15 mL) minced fresh hot chili pepper or dried chili flakes

1 Tbsp (15 mL) agave nectar or raw honey

2 Tbsp (30 mL) fish sauce or soy sauce

4 pink grapefruit

¼ cup (60 mL) chopped fresh mint

¼ cup (60 mL) cilantro

¼ cup (60 mL) chopped toasted almonds or other nuts

Heat oil in a small sauté pan over medium. Add shallots and chilis or chili flakes and cook, stirring, until shallots are golden. Transfer to a small bowl. Stir in agave nectar and fish or soy sauce.

With a sharp knife, cut peel and pith off grapefruit. Working over bowl containing shallot mixture to catch juice, cut out each segment between membranes. Spread grapefruit segments on a serving platter. Whisk shallot mixture well to combine ingredients thoroughly. Drizzle over grapefruit segments. Sprinkle mint, cilantro and almonds over top. Serve at room temperature.

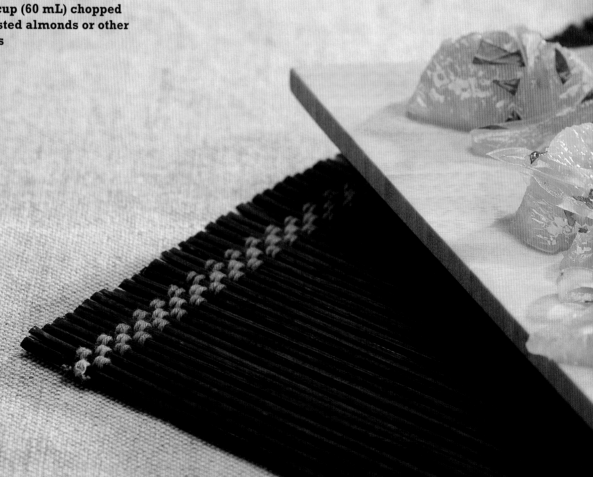

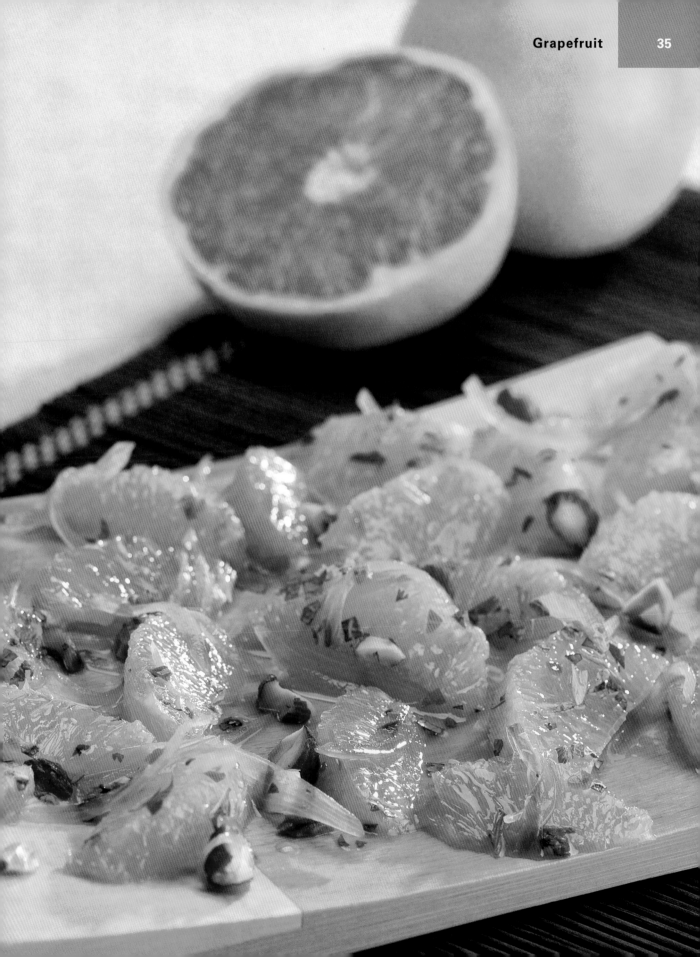

SUPER VEGGIES

Heal Thy Self with Vegetables

It's hard to argue with the health benefits of a diet rich in vegetables and fruits. Nutritionists may be able to point out a few drawbacks from eating too much meat, dairy or even fruit, but vegetables have consistently been held in high esteem—and for good reason. Vegetables are loaded with enough vitamins, minerals and other nutrients to make any mother smile when she sees her children eating them. The World Health Organization estimates that low intake of fruits and vegetables is responsible for about 19% of gastrointestinal cancer, 31% of ischemic heart disease and 11% of stroke worldwide. Overall, 2.7 million lives could be saved each year if fruit and vegetable consumption were increased. That's more that twice the number of lives lost globally from road traffic accidents.

The Inuit Paradox

But it isn't necessarily their nutrient content that makes vegetables so good for us. Ask traditional Inuit peoples who have thrived without eating a single vegetable in their lifetime. All vitamins and minerals can be found in meat products, including vitamin C. Researchers had long been baffled by the high incidence of scurvy among European Arctic explorers despite living on diets similar to the scurvy-free Inuit. This phenomenon could be explained by the Europeans' refusal to eat like the locals. Vitamin C is lost through cooking, so the natives would get their vitamin C from eating raw or minimally cooked meat like raw ringed seal liver or raw fatty whale skin (called muktuk). Explorers who didn't find the raw meat tempting could have gotten their vitamin C from the stomach contents of caribou, which was considered a delicacy for the Inuit. If that sounds absolutely scrumptious and you're thinking of adopting an Inuit diet, you should be more worried about an E. coli infection than about getting enough vitamin C. So please, cook your whale skin first.

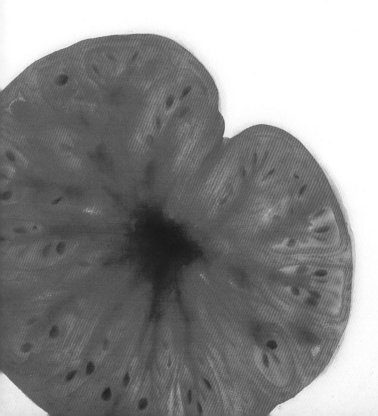

No-Nonsense Non-Nutrients

Vegetables are so good for us because they contain a diverse array of phytochemicals that have antioxidant, antibacterial, antifungal, antiviral, anti-inflammatory and anticarcinogenic activities that can prevent, halt or even reverse several diseases. No clinical study has ever shown that massive doses of vitamins or minerals can prevent cancer or other chronic diseases. Actually, mega-dosing of certain vitamins may actually increase your risk of developing certain cancers. Phytochemicals are made by plants to defend themselves against infection and damage caused by microbes and insects, or to enable them to survive in harsh environments. These same molecules impart their protective properties onto us, and several actually interfere with the sequence of events that trigger the formation of a tumour.

Because they are not considered essential in the respect that they do not cause deficiency symptoms if you do not consume them, phytochemicals are referred to as non-nutrients. This class includes dietary fibre: plant-based, indigestible carbohydrates that are important in the digestion and absorption of otherwise harmful substances. Dietary fibre produces healthy byproducts during bacterial fermentation in the colon and increases stool bulk, softens the stool, and shortens the transit time through the intestinal tract.

Consumption of high-fibre, phytochemical-rich vegetables may be one of the greatest weapons against cancer. Not all vegetables are created equal, however, so choose ones with more powerful punches. Dark green leafy vegetables and members of the cabbage family (broccoli, Brussels sprouts, cauliflower) should be headlining your dinner plate on a regular basis and are discussed separately.

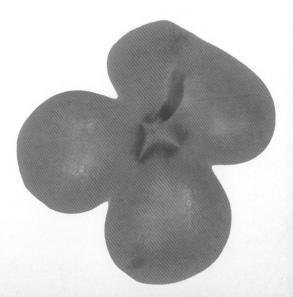

Asparagus

Asparagus has been used as a food and medicine for at least 20,000 years and appears in the world's oldest surviving cookbook, Apicius' 3rd century *De Re Coquinaria* (*On the Subject of Cooking*). The plant is notorious for producing malodorous urine (a polite way of saying stinky pee) because of sulphur-containing derivatives of asparagusic acid that are excreted in the urine. The onset of stinky pee is remarkably rapid, only 15 to 30 minutes after eating the asparagus. This diuretic characteristic is a result of the stimulation of renal activity and justifies the use of asparagus to treat hypertension. An excellent source of folate, potassium and fibre, asparagus is often served as a steamed, boiled or stir-fried vegetable side dish, often with hollandaise sauce, butter, olive oil or cheese. White asparagus, popular in many European countries, does not differ significantly from the green variety other than having a less bitter, more intensive taste, and containing less vitamin C.

Shaved Asparagus Salad with Oven-dried Tomatoes

Serves 4

1 tsp (5 mL) canola oil

4 medium shallots, quartered

1 bunch thick-stemmed asparagus

1 Tbsp (15 mL) extra-virgin olive oil

3 Tbsp (45 mL) balsamic vinegar

2 Tbsp (30 mL) chopped fresh thyme

½ tsp (2 mL) finely grated lemon zest

pinch each of sea salt and pepper

1 cup (250 mL) oven-dried tomatoes (see p. 51)

Heat oil in a small sauté pan over medium-low. Add shallots and cook, stirring, until softened and just beginning to turn golden. Remove from heat and set aside to cool to room temperature.

Snap off bottom ends of asparagus at their natural breaking point by bending lower part of stalks. Discard bottoms. Cut tips from asparagus. Drop into boiling salted water and cook for 2 minutes. Remove from water with a slotted spoon and transfer to an ice water bath to refresh. Drop stalks into boiling water and cook for 30 seconds. Transfer to same ice water bath. Once they are cool, use a vegetable peeler to slice asparagus stalks into ribbons.

Combine oil, vinegar, thyme, lemon zest, salt and pepper in small bowl. Whisk until well combined.

Divide asparagus ribbons among 4 plates. Scatter shallots, asparagus tips and oven-dried tomatoes over ribbons. Drizzle with dressing and serve immediately.

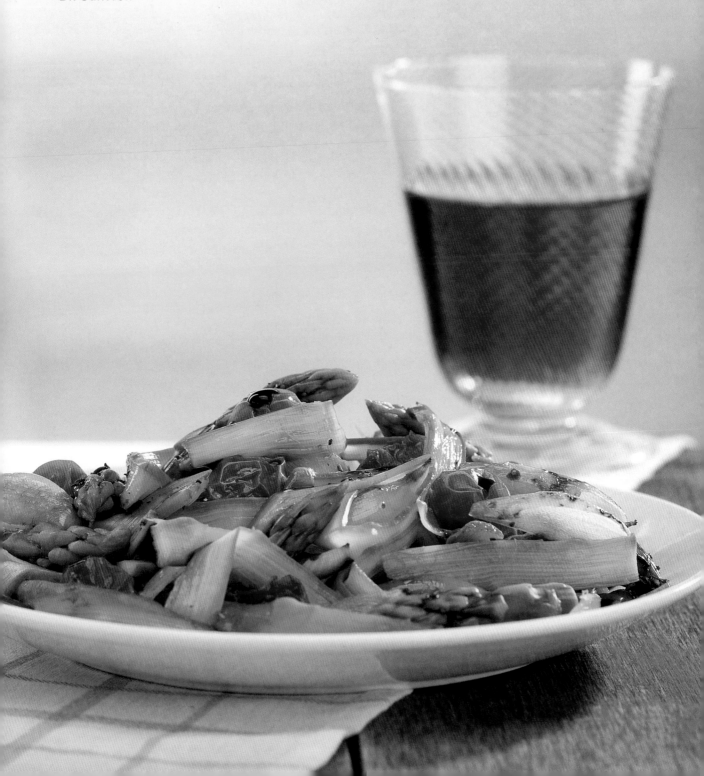

*The colors of a fresh garden salad are so extraordinary,
no painter's pallet can duplicate nature's artistry.*

—Dr. SunWolf

Asparagus Bisque

Serves 4

1 bunch of asparagus

3 cups (750 mL) vegetable stock

1 bouquet garni (see Tip)

2 tsp (10 mL) canola oil

1 medium white onion, chopped

½ leek, white and pale green parts only, chopped

1 clove garlic, minced

1 cup (250 mL) diced, peeled potato, in ½ in (1 cm) pieces

Trim root ends of asparagus and reserve trimmings. Cut about 1½ in (3 cm) from tips of asparagus and reserve. Chop stalks into 1 in (2 cm) pieces. Set aside. Bring stock to a simmer in a large saucepan. Add asparagus trimmings and *bouquet garni*. Simmer for 30 minutes.

Meanwhile, heat oil in a second large saucepan over medium-low. Add onion, leek and garlic. Cook, stirring occasionally, until softened, about 5 minutes. Add potatoes. Strain vegetable stock from first pot into second, discarding asparagus trimmings. Bring to a simmer over medium-high. Reduce heat to medium. Cover and simmer until potatoes are tender, about 5 minutes. Add asparagus stalks. Simmer until asparagus is just tender, about 4 minutes. Purée in a blender or with a hand blender. Pass through a fine-mesh strainer into a bowl.

Cut asparagus tips in half lengthwise. Blanch quickly in boiling water until tender-crisp, 1 to 2 minutes depending on thickness. Ladle soup into bowls. Garnish with asparagus tips. (Can be served hot or cold, but if serving chilled, soup should be set into a larger bowl partly filled with ice immediately after straining.)

Tip

A bouquet garni is a bundle of herbs that is removed from a dish before eating. To make a bouquet garni, stick 2 whole cloves into a 4 inch (10 cm) piece of celery. Tie celery with 4 stems of fresh parsley (without leaves), 4 sprigs of fresh thyme and 2 bay leaves.

This soup can also be made using mostly asparagus trimmings, if you save them in your freezer; the colour will be a little less vibrant, but the taste will be the same. Just substitute the stalks with more trimmings, cook and purée as directed.

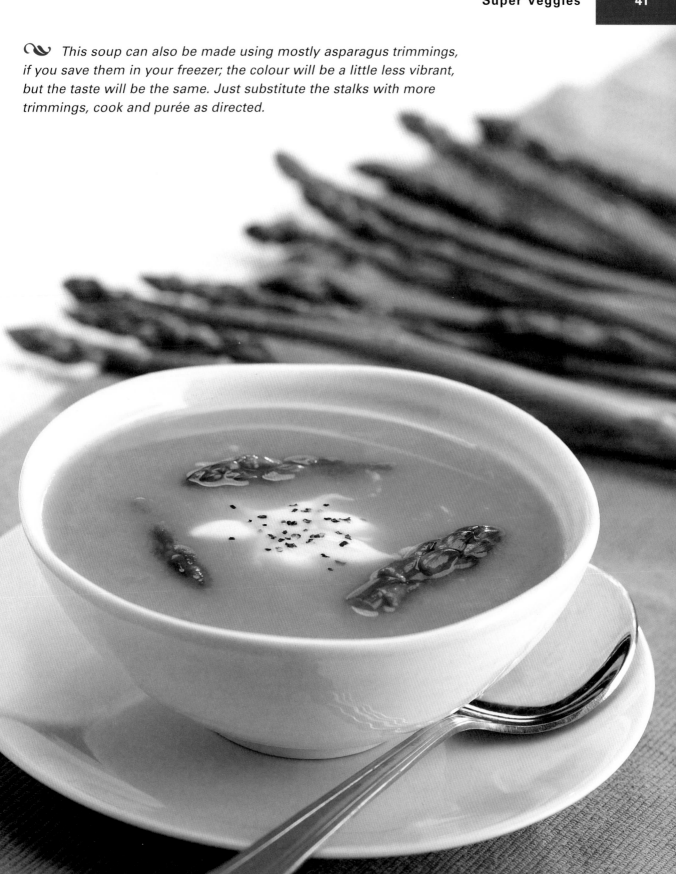

Avocado

Avocado is a tree native to Mexico and is an example of an "evolutionary anachronism." Its large fleshy fruit was adapted to be consumed by large, now-extinct mammals such as giant ground sloths or elephant-like gomphotheres, who would then excrete the seed in their dung, ready to sprout. Today most avocados are propagated by grafting. Avocados are incredible for your health and should not be avoided by those who are fat phobic. The fat content is mostly from healthy monounsaturated fats and does not contribute to weight gain. Avocados contain more than 25 essential nutrients and have 60% more potassium than bananas. Studies show that high avocado intake lowers blood levels of low-density lipoproteins (LDL) and triglycerides, and increases high-density lipoproteins (HDL). The flesh also contains phytochemicals that have potent anti-inflammatory properties and can reduce the risk of inflammatory and degenerative diseases. Enjoy avocados guilt-free!

Creamy Avocado Mango Dressing

Makes 1 cup (250 mL)

1 avocado, chopped

1 mango, chopped

2 Tbsp (30 mL) chopped fresh basil

2 Tbsp (30 mL) lime juice

1 Tbsp (15 mL) minced ginger

pinch each of sea salt and pepper

Combine all ingredients in a blender. Process until smooth. Drizzle over salad or steamed, roasted or grilled veggies.

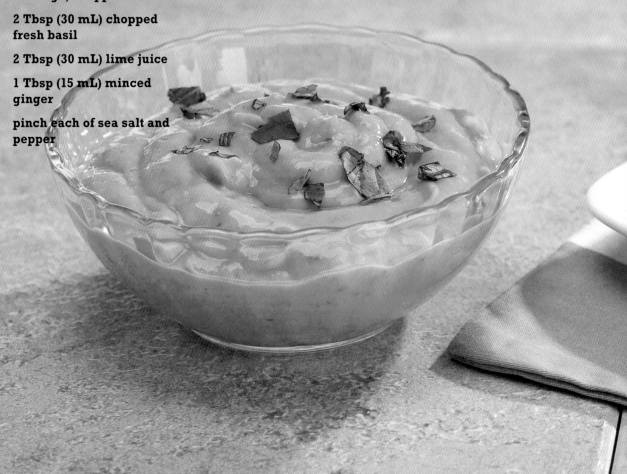

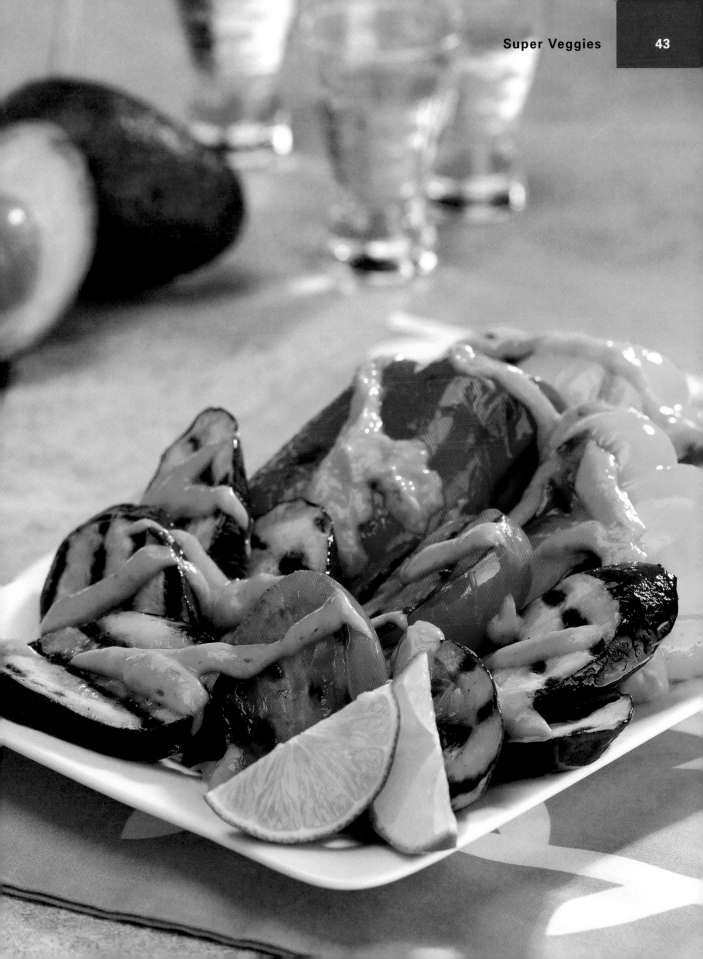

Grilled Avocado with Strawberry Papaya Salsa

Serves 4

1 cup (250 mL) diced papaya, cut in ½ in (1 cm) pieces

1 cup (250 mL) diced strawberries, cut in ½ in (1 cm) pieces

1 Tbsp (15 mL) balsamic vinegar

⅓ cup (75 mL) orange juice

2 Tbsp (30 mL) lime juice

¼ cup (60 mL) canola oil

¼ cup (60 mL) raw honey

4 firm ripe avocados

Combine papaya, strawberries, vinegar, orange and lime juices in a medium bowl. Cover and refrigerate for at least 30 minutes to combine flavours.

Preheat grill to medium-high. In a separate small bowl, combine oil and honey. Halve, pit and peel avocados. Cut lengthwise into ¾ in (1.5 cm) thick slices. Brush oil and honey mixture onto all sides of avocado slices (you will not use all of mixture). Cook avocado slices on a well-greased grill until well marked, about 3 to 4 minutes per side (use a spatula to turn avocado slices rather than tongs, which would break them). Divide avocado slices among 4 plates and spoon salsa over.

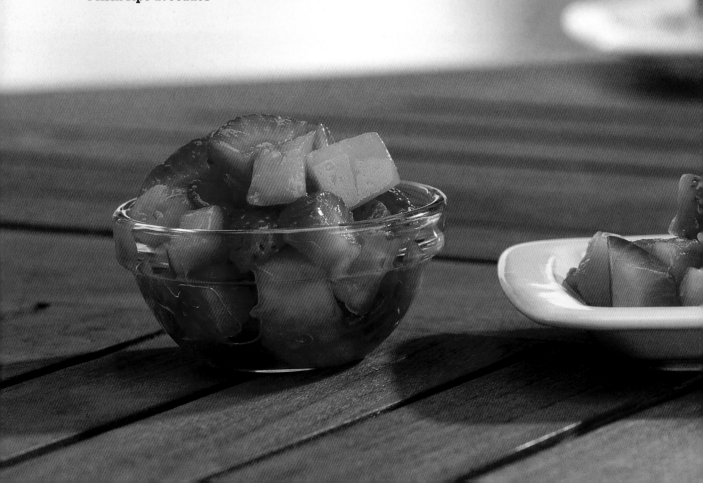

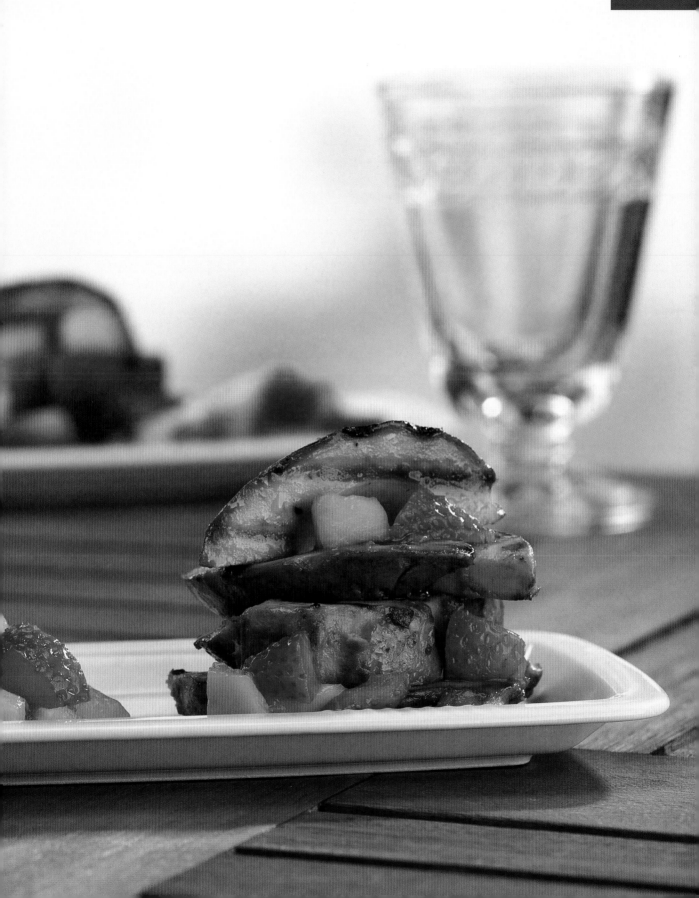

Peppers

Peppers come in a rainbow of colours and are loaded with nutrients and bioactive phytochemicals. A great source of vitamin C, folate and B vitamins, they also contain carotenoids that give them their vibrant colours. Red bell peppers contain more nutrients than the green varieties, and they also contain lycopene, an antioxidant carotenoid that has been studied for its preventative properties against cancer and cardiovascular disease. Hot chili peppers contain capsaicin as the active ingredient, an irritant that produces the familiar burning sensation that can make your eyes water. Besides keeping muggers at bay when in the form of pepper spray, capsaicin can also inhibit the growth of prostate cancer cells, provide pain relief, relieve congestion, decrease inflammation, soothe irritable bowel syndrome, burn fat by increasing your metabolism and reduce LDL cholesterol. Careful not to eat hot peppers in large quantities or touch other areas of your body after handling them: painful exposure to hot peppers is among the most common plant-related complaints presented to poison centres.

Smoky Fresh Pepper Salsa

Makes 4 cups (1 L)

6 Roma tomatoes, cut into ¼ in (0.5 cm) dice

2 red peppers, cut into ¼ in (0.5 cm) dice

1 yellow pepper, cut into ¼ in (0.5 cm) dice

1 red onion, cut into ¼ in (0.5 cm) dice

1 bunch green onions, thinly sliced

4 chipotle peppers in adobo sauce, finely chopped

½ cup (125 mL) lime juice

1 bunch cilantro, chopped

2 cloves garlic, minced

salt and pepper

Combine tomatoes, peppers, onions, chipotles, lime juice, cilantro and garlic in a medium bowl. Add salt and pepper to taste. Cover and refrigerate for at least 1 hour before serving to allow flavours to combine.

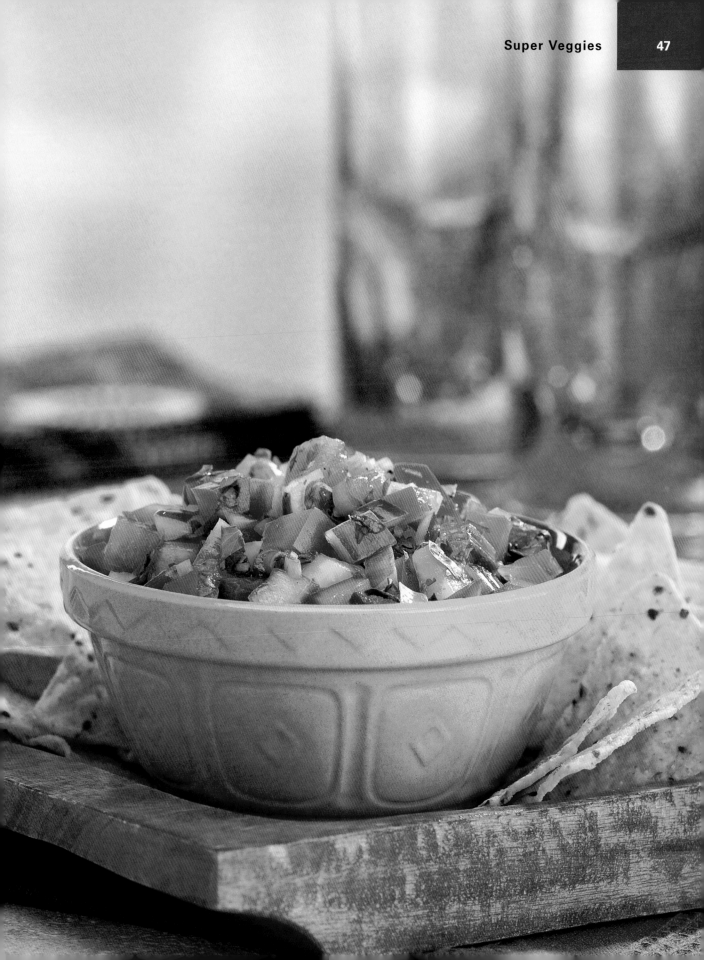

Roasted Red Pepper Sauce

Makes about 1¹/₂ cups (375 mL)

1 tsp (5 mL) canola oil

½ small onion, chopped

3 cloves garlic, minced

3 roasted red peppers

1 cup (250 mL) vegetable stock

¼ cup (60 mL) loosely packed chopped fresh basil

¼ tsp (1 mL) sea salt

½ tsp (2 mL) pepper

Heat oil in a small sauté pan on medium. Add onion and garlic and cook, stirring, until softened and starting to turn golden. Transfer to a blender.

Add roasted peppers, stock, basil, salt and pepper to blender. Purée until smooth. Warm over medium-low heat to serve over fish, vegetable, pasta or grain dishes.

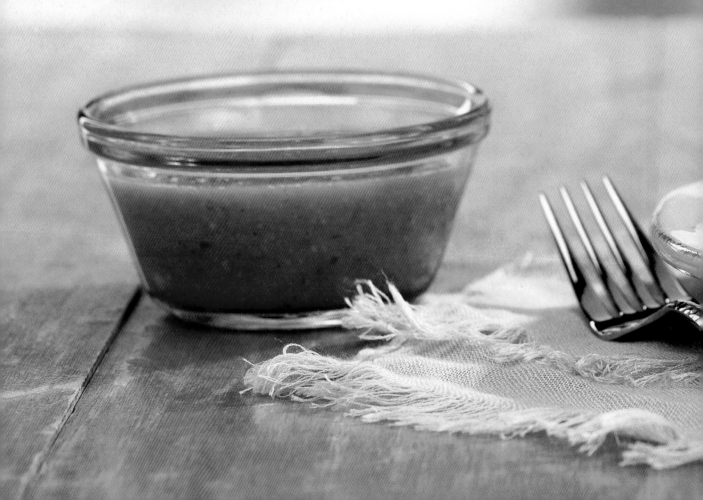

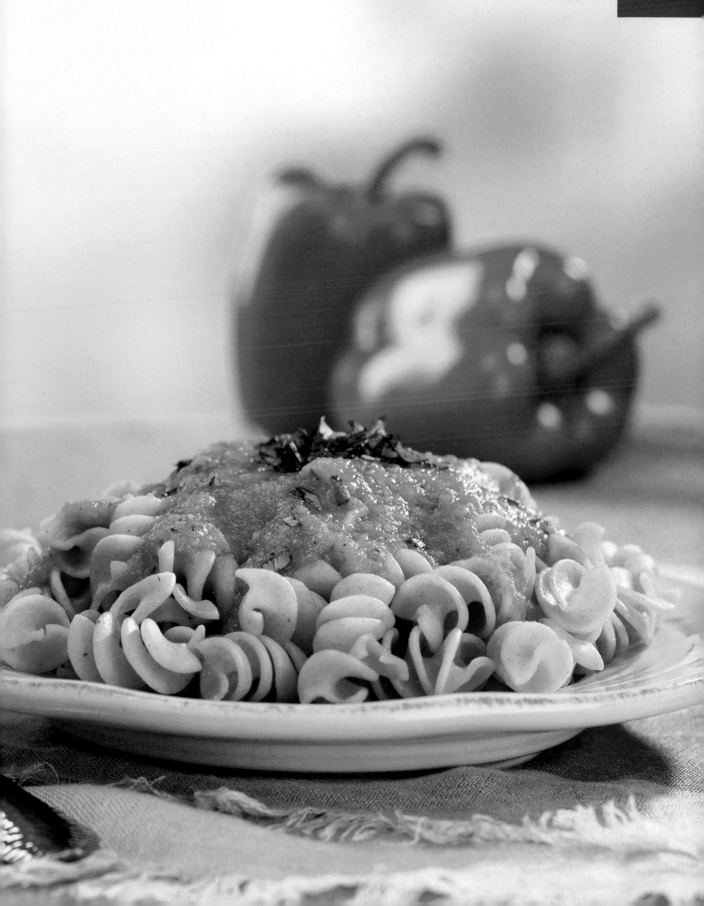

Tomatoes

Like peppers, tomatoes belong to the nightshade family (Solanaceae), a group that contains the malevolently poisonous deadly nightshade, henbane, jimsonweed, mandrake and tobacco. Perhaps it was because of this association that the tomato was considered unfit for eating when it was first introduced to Britain and its colonies in the 16th century. By the mid-18th century though, tomatoes were eaten on a daily basis. They are particularly rich in lycopene, which is apparently absorbed more readily in a processed form, such as tomato paste, stewed tomatoes and tomato juices. This could be used as an excuse to help yourself to an extra serving of spaghetti sauce! It's wise to eat tomatoes and red peppers every day. As little as 10 milligrams of lycopene (the amount found in one large tomato or one 12 oz (340 g) glass of tomato juice or sauce) was found to prevent osteoporosis, a disease of bone deterioration.

Two Tomato Sauce

Makes 3$\frac{1}{2}$ cups (875 mL)

$\frac{1}{2}$ cup (125 mL) packed sun-dried tomatoes (look for dry ones, not oil-packed, or use Oven-dried Tomatoes, see facing page)

1 cup (250 mL) boiling water

1 Tbsp (15 mL) canola oil

2 cups (500 mL) chopped onion

6 cloves garlic, minced

32 oz (900 mL) can whole tomatoes, with liquid

$\frac{1}{2}$ cup (125 mL) red wine

2 bay leaves

$\frac{1}{2}$ tsp (2 mL) sea salt

1 tsp (5 mL) pepper

$\frac{1}{4}$ cup chopped fresh basil

$\frac{1}{4}$ cup chopped fresh oregano

Soak sun-dried tomatoes in boiling water in a small bowl for 30 minutes. Drain over a bowl, reserving liquid. Chop soaked tomatoes coarsely.

Meanwhile, heat oil in a medium saucepan over medium-low. Add onion and garlic. Cook, stirring occasionally, until softened, about 5 minutes. Add canned tomatoes and their liquid, chopped tomatoes and their soaking liquid, red wine, bay leaves, salt and pepper. Cook uncovered, stirring occasionally to break up tomatoes, for about 30 minutes. Remove and discard bay leaves and add basil and oregano. Purée with a hand blender or in a blender until smooth.

Oven-dried Tomatoes

2 lbs (1 kg) cherry or Roma tomatoes

sea salt

Preheat oven to 150° F (65° C) or its lowest setting and oil
2 baking sheets. Cut tomatoes in half. Sprinkle a little salt
on cut sides. Arrange, cut side down, on sheets. Bake until
darkened in colour and dry to the touch but still flexible,
about 6 to 8 hours. Make sure they are fully dried, or they
will mould in storage. Store for up to 3 months sealed in
plastic bags or glass jars out of direct light.

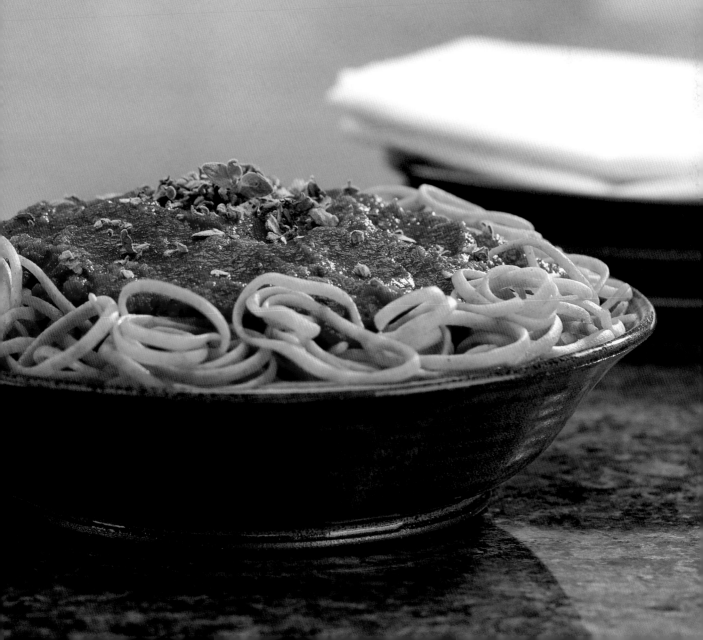

Spicy Gazpacho

Serves 4

4 Roma tomatoes, *divided*

1 clove garlic, minced

½ tsp (2 mL) salt, plus more to taste

2 cups (500 mL) tomato juice, *divided*

½ English cucumber, cut in ¼ in (0.5 cm) dice, *divided*

½ cup (125 mL) diced yellow bell pepper, cut in ¼ in (0.5 cm) pieces, *divided*

½ medium red onion, cut in a ¼ in (0.5 cm) dice

2 Tbsp (30 mL) chopped fresh cilantro

2 Tbsp (30 mL) chopped fresh basil

1½ Tbsp (22 mL) lime juice

½ green onion, minced

2 tsp (10 mL) minced hot chili pepper

pepper to taste

1 firm-ripe avocado, cut in a ¼ in (0.5 cm) dice

Cut tomatoes in half crosswise. Squeeze out and discard seeds. Cut tomato flesh into ¼ in (0.5 cm) dice.

Mash garlic and salt on work surface and form into a paste using side of a knife.

Place ½ cup (125 mL) of tomato juice and half each of tomatoes, cucumber and bell pepper in blender. Purée until smooth. Transfer to a large bowl. Add remaining tomatoes, cucumber and bell pepper, as well as onion, cilantro, basil, lime juice, green onion, chili pepper and garlic paste to bowl. Stir until well combined. Transfer ½ cup (125 mL) to blender. Add ¾ cup (180 mL) tomato juice to blender. Purée until smooth. Transfer back to bowl and stir until well combined. Thin to desired consistency with remaining tomato juice. Add salt and pepper to taste. Cover and refrigerate for at least 2 hours up to overnight before serving. Divide among 4 serving bowls and sprinkle with diced avocado.

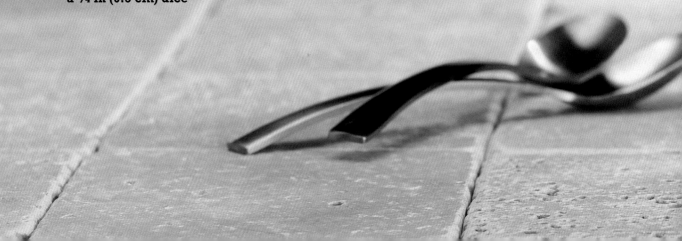

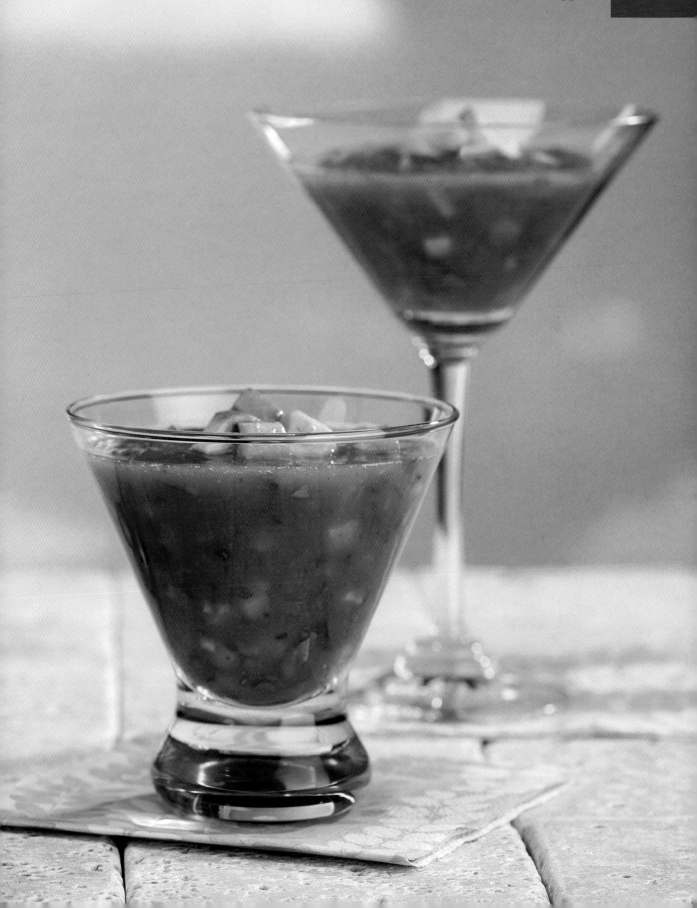

LEAFY GREENS

Leaf It to the Experts

Spinach, dandelion, kale, watercress, chard, arugula, bok choy and many others, belong to a class of vegetables called leafy greens, potherbs or salad greens. Edible leaves have been part of the human diet since we first appeared on Earth. They are, calorie for calorie, perhaps the most concentrated source of vitamins and minerals of any food. They are especially rich in vitamins A, C and K, calcium, potassium, iron and manganese. They are brimming with dietary fibre and have very little impact on blood glucose, which is perfect for diabetics or those following a low-carb diet. And like chocolates and sunglasses, the darker, the better. Dark green leaves contain much more nutrients and phytochemicals than lighter ones. Lettuce for example does not contain much more than water, yet it is the most frequently eaten leaf in the U.S., consumed as a garnish in burgers and tacos.

It's Not Easy Being Leafy Dark Green

People are unfortunately not consuming nearly as many leafy greens as they should be, and the 2006 *E. coli* strain O157:H7 outbreak in the U.S. didn't help matters. Because many leafy greens grow close to the ground, they can become contaminated with soil, dirty water, improperly composted manure or by wild and domestic animals. Bacteria can also be transferred during and after harvest from handling, storing and transporting. Because they're often eaten raw, leafy greens can be a source of food-borne illness. To ensure that your leafy greens are clean, choose crisp leaves that are not wilted or brown. Remove the outer leaves and make sure all the dirt is gone. Wash the leaves under fresh, cool running water, not in

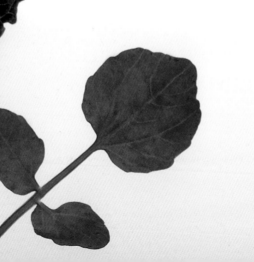
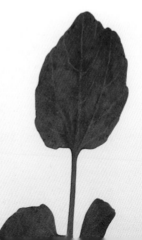

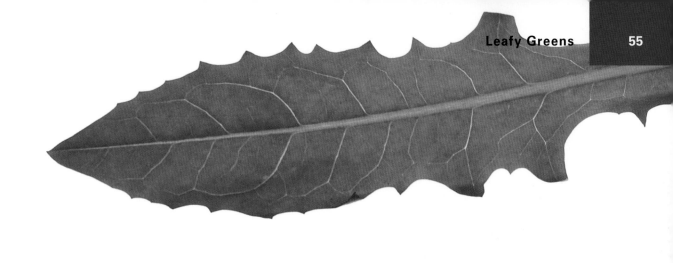

a sink full of standing water. Ready-to-eat, bagged, pre-washed leafy greens don't need to be washed again, but pre-cut greens sold in open bags or containers should be. And of course, wash your hands before handling your food. The majority of contaminations are usually spread by the unwashed hands of food handler or consumer who is all.

Take It or Leaf It

Leafy dark green vegetables are a crucial part of a healthy diet, so try to sneak them in your diet as often as possible. Other than in salads, add them to omelets and pasta sauces, and pile them into your sandwiches and burgers. Probably the sneakiest way to eat them is to include them in your smoothies. Despite what Kermit says, it's not that hard being green.

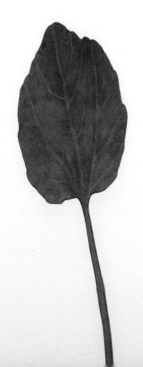

Dandelions

Dandelions may be considered unwanted weeds on your lawn, but you definitely want them in your salads (as long as they have not been treated with herbicides). The leaves are rather bitter, so they are usually blanched to make them more palatable when bought commercially. Dandelions have long been used in traditional medicines as an effective diuretic. They contain high levels of potassium salts needed to replenish any that are lost when diuretics are normally used. There is also evidence that they possess anti-inflammatory properties that may be helpful in treating urinary tract infections in women.

Asian Stir-fried Greens

Serves 4

1 Tbsp (15 mL) canola oil

2 cloves garlic, minced

2 tsp (10 mL) minced fresh ginger

3 Tbsp (45 mL) rice vinegar

2 Tbsp (30 mL) soy sauce

2 tsp (10 mL) agave nectar

4 cups (1 L) Swiss chard, trimmed

4 cups (1 L) dandelion leaves, trimmed

4 cups (1 L) watercress, trimmed

1 tsp (5 mL) sesame oil

Heat oil in a wok over medium-high heat. Add garlic and cook, stirring constantly, until just starting to colour. Add ginger and cook, stirring constantly, until fragrant. Stir in rice vinegar, soy sauce and agave nectar. Add Swiss chard and cook, stirring, for 2 minutes. Add dandelion leaves and watercress and cook, stirring, until wilted, about 2 minutes more.

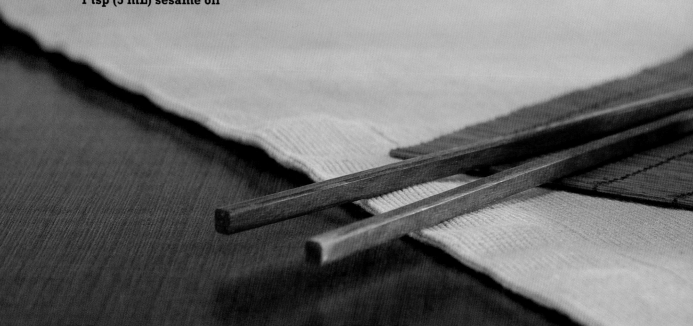

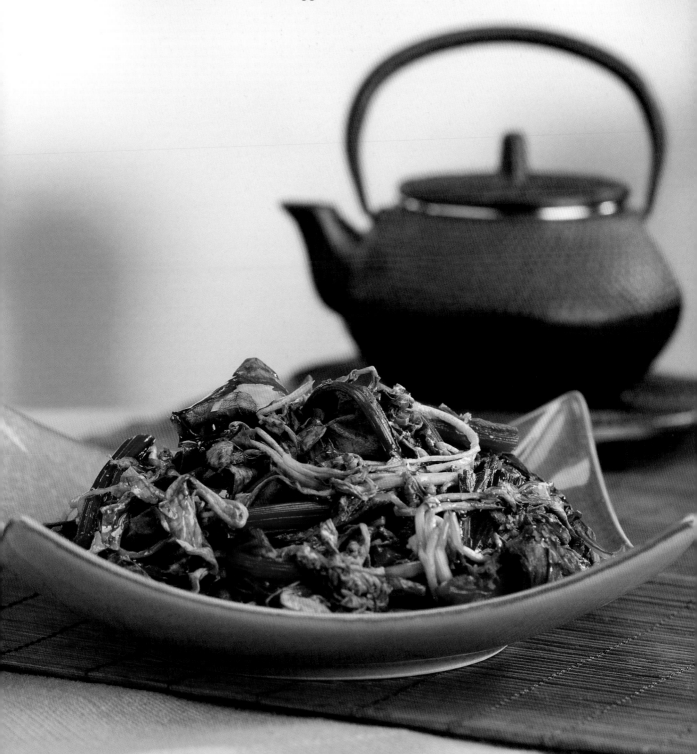

∾ *Greens are the No. 1 food you can eat regularly to help improve your health.*

—Jill Nussinow, MS, RD, author of *The Veggie Queen*

Dandelion with Radish and Fennel in Hazelnut Mustard Vinaigrette

Serves 4

1 small shallot, minced

½ tsp (2 mL) salt

1 Tbsp (15 mL) grainy Dijon mustard

1 Tbsp (15 mL) red wine vinegar

¼ tsp (1 mL) pepper

¼ cup (60 mL) hazelnut oil

4 cups (1 L) loosely packed dandelion leaves, trimmed of tough stems if large, cut crosswise into 2 in (5 cm) wide strips

1 bulb fennel, trimmed, cored and thinly sliced

1 bunch radishes, trimmed and thinly sliced

Mix together shallot and salt with side of a knife to form a paste. Transfer to a small bowl and add mustard, vinegar and pepper. Whisk thoroughly. Slowly add oil, whisking constantly, until emulsified.

Combine dandelion leaves, fennel and radish in a large bowl. Drizzle with dressing and toss to coat. Serve immediately.

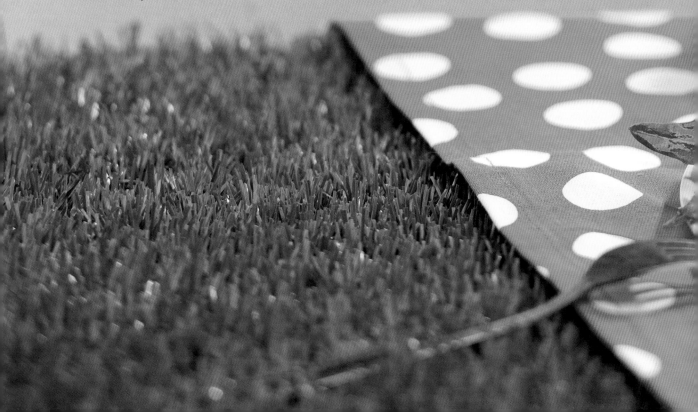

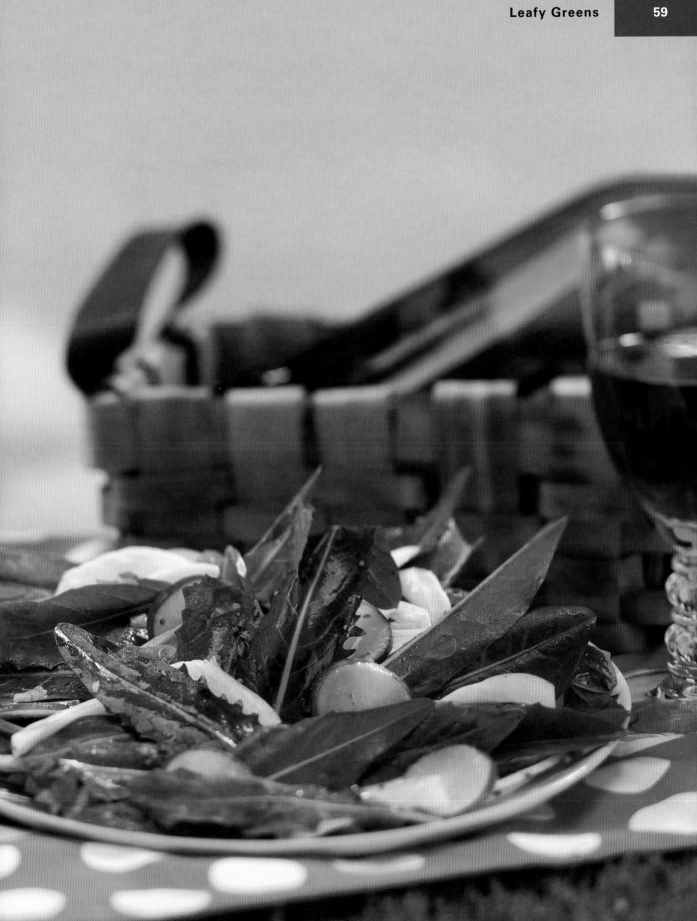

Kale

Kale is particularly good for your health. It is the same species as cabbage, broccoli, collard greens and Brussels sprouts, and therefore contains the same cancer-fighting phytochemicals such as sulforaphane and indole-3-carbinol. These compounds boost DNA repair and block the formation of tumours. Make sure to conserve these compounds and other vitamins and minerals by steaming, microwaving or stir-frying the leaves, rather than boiling, which causes significant loss.

Gingered Kale and Apple Slaw

Serves 4

1 lb (500 g) decorative curly kale, trimmed of tough ribs

2 Tbsp (30 mL) coarse sea salt

2 Tbsp (30 mL) rice vinegar

1 small shallot, minced

1 Tbsp (15 mL) minced ginger

2 tsp (10 mL) raw honey

1 tsp (5 mL) finely grated lemon zest

1 Tbsp (15 mL) canola oil

½ Tbsp (7 mL) sesame oil

sea salt and pepper

1 cup (250 mL) julienned apple (skin on)

Working in batches, stack kale leaves and cut diagonally into ¼ in (0.5 cm) wide strips. Transfer to a large bowl. Sprinkle with salt and toss to coat. Place a plate on top and add a weight on top of plate (such as a saucepan of water). Let stand 15 minutes. Toss. Replace plate and weight and let stand another 15 minutes. Drain and rinse several times. Transfer to a salad spinner and dry as much as possible.

Combine rice vinegar and shallot and let stand 15 minutes. Add ginger, honey and lemon zest and stir to combine. Drizzle in both oils, whisking constantly until well combined. Season to taste with salt and pepper.

Combine kale and apple in a large bowl. Drizzle with dressing and toss to coat. Serve immediately or cover and refrigerate for up to 2 hours before serving.

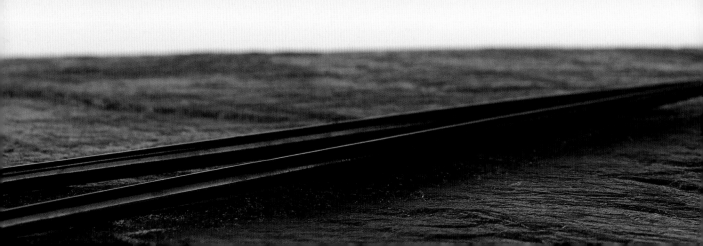

The apple is another fruit that has been given superfood status. It ranks second among popular fruit for the highest levels of antioxidants (beaten only by cranberries) and is high in quercetin, a flavonoid that has anticancer properties. It is also one of the best sources of boron, which is vital for building bone and can help prevent osteoporosis.

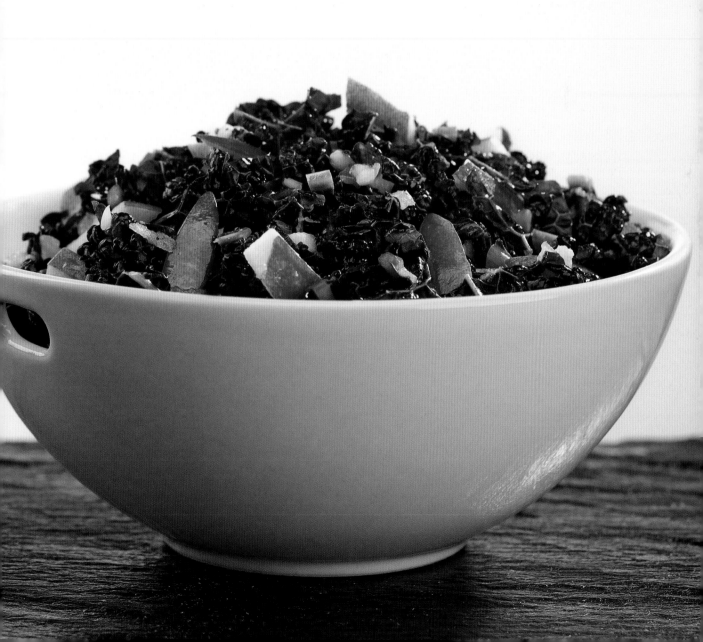

Baked Kale with Sweet Potato

Serves 4

1½ lbs (680 g) curly kale, trimmed of tough ribs

1 Tbsp (15 mL) canola oil

2 cloves garlic, minced

1½ lbs (680 g) sweet potato, cut into ¼ in (0.5 cm) slices

½ cup (125 mL) water

¼ cup (60 mL) lime juice

1 Tbsp (15 mL) chopped fresh rosemary

1 tsp (5 mL) finely grated lime zest

½ tsp (2 mL) sea salt

pepper to taste

Preheat oven to 350° F (175° C). Working in batches, stack kale leaves and cut diagonally into strips ½ in (1 cm) wide.

Heat canola oil in a large sauté pan over medium-low. Add garlic and cook, stirring, until fragrant and light golden, about 4 minutes. Add sweet potatoes and stir to coat. Add kale, water and lime juice. Bring to a boil. Stir in rosemary, lime zest and salt. Transfer to large casserole dish. Cover and bake, stirring occasionally, until sweet potatoes are just tender, about 30 minutes. Add pepper to taste. Serve immediately or at room temperature.

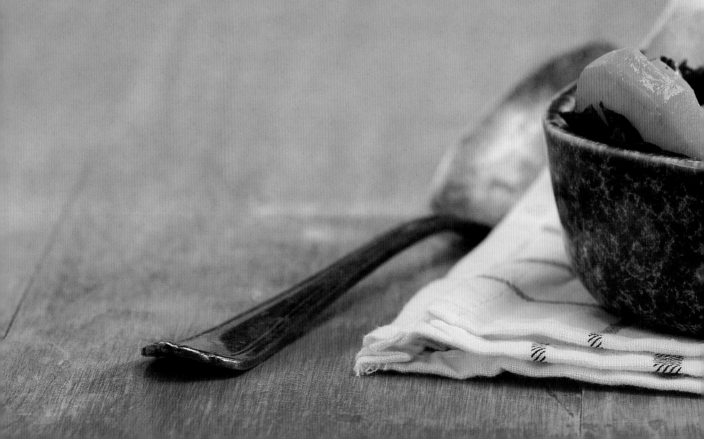

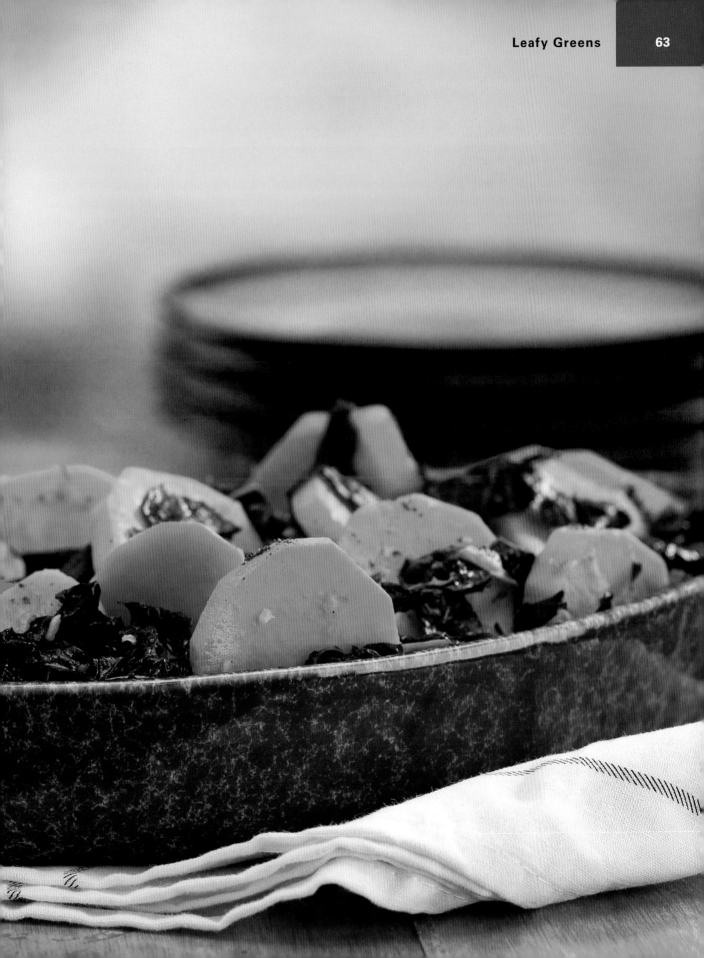

Spinach

Spinach is an excellent source of vitamin A, occurring as its precursor beta-carotene, which is a powerful antioxidant that helps reduce the risk of developing cataracts, and prevents heart disease and cancer. It is also rich in other carotenoids, namely lutein and zeaxanthin, which help prevent age-related macular degeneration. Spinach is a rich source of iron; however, only a fraction of the mineral is available for absorption because it is usually bound to oxalates that occur naturally in the leaves. Oxalates also tightly bind calcium, allowing only 5% to be available for absorption. Those worried about bone health should not be too concerned though: 1 cup (250 mL) of steamed spinach provides over 1000% of the RDA of vitamin K needed to maintain bone strength and density. Vitamin K is also essential for carboxylation of proteins, a process that prevents calcium build-up in tissues and also fights atherosclerosis and stroke. If eaten raw, spinach is an excellent source of vitamin C.

Spinach and Artichoke Dip

Makes about 3 cups (750 mL)

$1\frac{1}{2}$ cups (375 mL) firm silken tofu

3 Tbsp (45 mL) lemon juice

1 head of roasted garlic

2 cloves garlic, minced

$\frac{1}{2}$ tsp (2 mL) apple cider vinegar

$\frac{1}{2}$ tsp (2 mL) sea salt plus more to taste

pepper to taste

1 to 2 pinches of powdered kelp or spirulina

Tabasco sauce to taste

1 bunch spinach, cut crosswise into $\frac{1}{2}$ in (1 cm) wide strips

$\frac{1}{2}$ small jar of artichoke hearts, rinsed and drained, cut into $\frac{1}{8}$ths

Combine tofu, lemon juice, roasted garlic, fresh garlic, vinegar, salt, kelp or spirulina and Tabasco in a food processor. Process until smooth. Transfer to a medium casserole, and stir in spinach and artichoke hearts. Season with pepper. Cover and bake in preheated 350° F (175° C) oven until warmed through, about 20 to 30 minutes.

We've all heard of Popeye the sailor who developed superhuman strength after downing a can of spinach. As the story goes, Popeye's creator, Elzie Crisler Segar, chose the vegetable because of its high iron content after a misplaced decimal in an 1870 publication led to a popular belief that spinach had 10 times more iron than it actually contains. The error was discovered in 1937, but it was too late: Popeye was already telling every child and parent to eat their spinach, leading to an increase in the crop's sales and a significant impact on public health nutrition policy. Recently, however, the entire misplaced decimal story has been debunked. In truth, Segar chose spinach as the source of Popeye's powers because of its vitamin A content, which scientists in the 1920s discovered could significantly improve a child's nutritional status.

That spinach is high in vitamin C is ironic considering that Popeye may have been suffering from scurvy, which was relatively common in sailors. The protrusion of one eye may have been the result of a hemorrhage behind the eyeball caused by scurvy, and the way his pipe juts up in front of his face may be because he lost all his teeth and is holding it between his upper and lower gums. Segar claims that the character was modelled after a coal miner friend of his, but who says that miners didn't get scurvy as well?

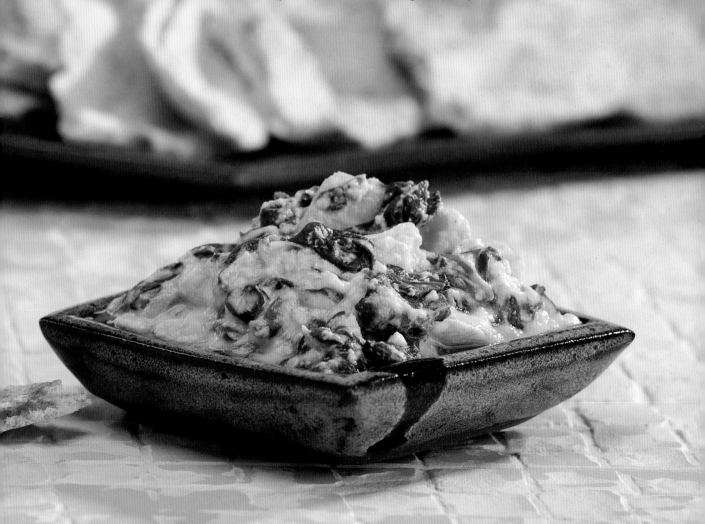

Savoury Tomato Vegetable Soup with Spinach

Serves 4

1 Tbsp (15 mL) canola oil

½ cup (125 mL) diced onion, cut in ½ inch (1 cm) pieces

2 cloves of garlic, minced

½ cup (125 mL) diced carrot cut in ½ inch (1 cm) pieces

1 stalk celery, cut in ½ inch (1 cm) dice

½ medium zucchini, cut in ½ inch (1 cm) dice

1 x 14 oz (398 mL) can crushed tomatoes

2½ cups (625 mL) vegetable stock

4 Tbsp (60 mL) chopped fresh basil, *divided*

4 Tbsp (60 mL) chopped flat-leaf parsley, *divided*

¼ tsp (1 mL) sea salt

¼ tsp (1 mL) pepper

1½ cups (375 mL) chopped fresh spinach

Heat oil in a large saucepan over medium. Add onion and garlic. Cook, stirring, until onion has softened, about 5 minutes. Add carrot, celery and zucchini and cook, stirring until softened, about 10 minutes. Add crushed tomatoes, stock, 2 Tbsp (30 mL) each of basil and parsley, and salt and pepper. Bring to a boil, then cover and reduce heat.

Simmer, stirring occasionally, for about 30 minutes. Stir in spinach, cover again and cook another 10 minutes. Adjust seasoning with salt and pepper to taste, stir in remaining basil and parsley and serve immediately.

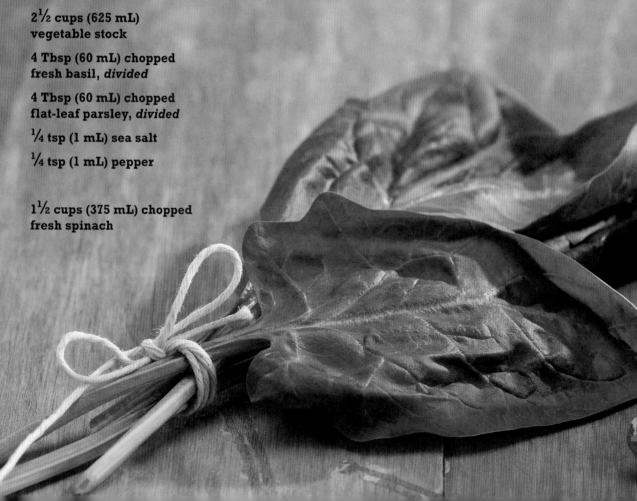

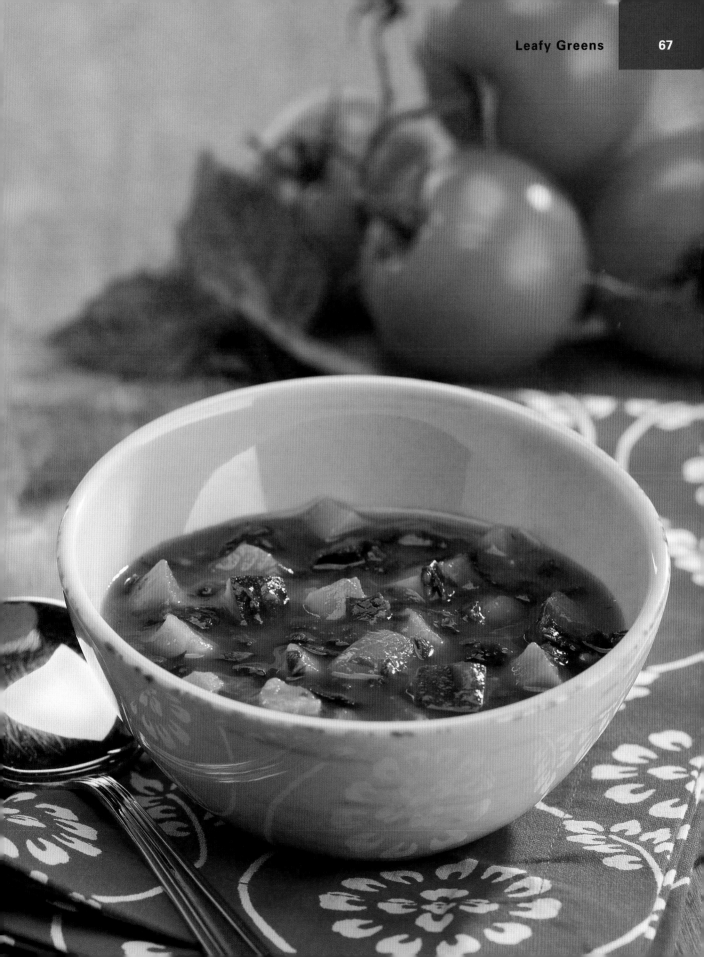

Watercress

One of the oldest known leaf vegetables consumed by humans, watercress is among the best plant sources of iodine. This trace mineral is crucial for proper functioning of the thyroid gland, which uses it to produce thyroid hormones. Low levels of these hormones cause extreme fatigue, goiter, depression, weight gain and low body temperatures. An iodine deficiency is the leading cause of preventable mental retardation. The addition of iodine to salt has largely eliminated this problem in developed countries, but it remains a serious public health problem in the rest of the world. Like other leafy greens, watercress has been found to significantly reduce DNA damage and increase the ability of cells to resist further damage caused by free radicals. Research suggests that it may be able to inhibit the growth of lung and breast cancer.

Sautéed Watercress and Chard with Hot Pepper Vinegar

Serves 4

½ cup (125 mL) apple cider vinegar

1 Tbsp (15 mL) crushed red pepper flakes

1 Tbsp (15 mL) canola oil

4 cloves garlic, minced

4 cups (1 L) watercress, trimmed

4 cups (1 L) Swiss chard, cut crosswise into 2 in (5 cm) wide strips

Combine vinegar and pepper flakes in a small bowl. Cover and let stand overnight. Strain and discard solids.

Heat oil in a large sauté pan over medium. Add garlic and cook, stirring, until fragrant, about 1 minute. Add watercress and chard. Cook, stirring occasionally to bring cooked leaves up toward top, until leaves are just wilted, about 5 to 7 minutes. Sprinkle 2 Tbsp (30 mL) of hot pepper vinegar over and toss to coat. Serve immediately with remaining pepper vinegar on side.

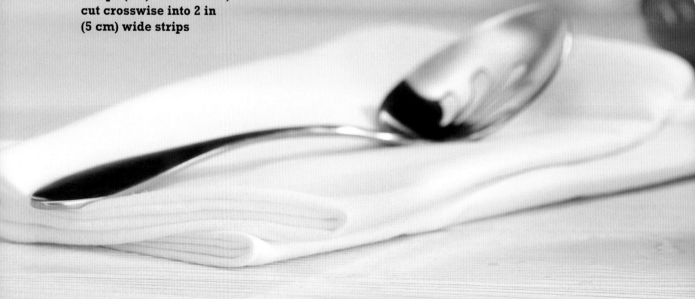

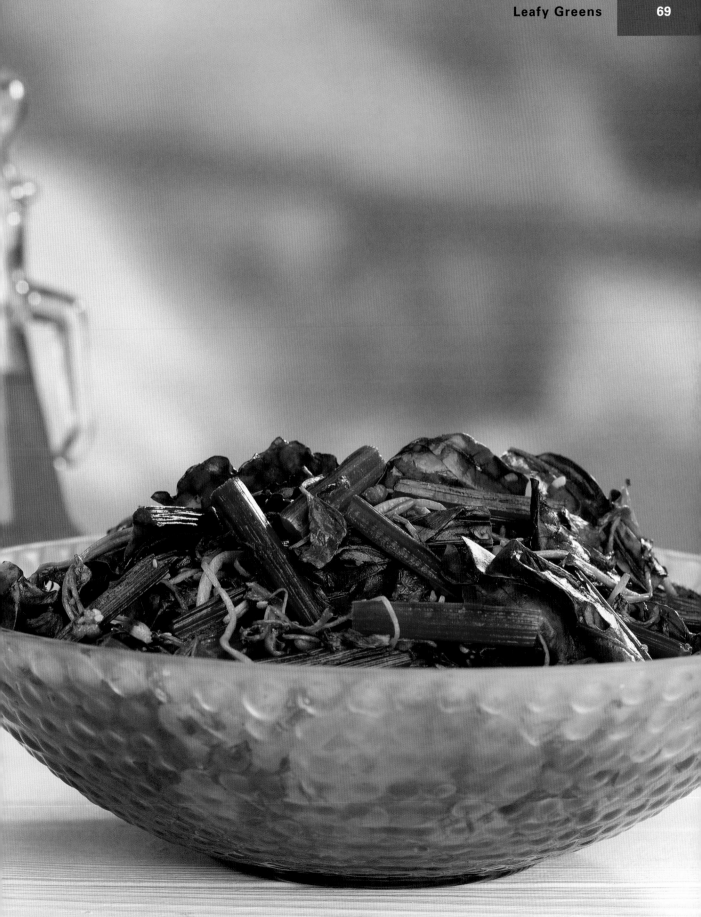

Watercress and Avocado Salad

Serves 6

¼ cup (60 mL) unseasoned rice vinegar

1 Tbsp (15 mL) grated sweet onion such as Vidalia or Walla Walla (use large holes of a box grater)

¼ cup (60 mL) finely grated peeled Gala apple (use small holes of a box grater)

4 tsp (20 mL) soy sauce

1 tsp (5 mL) raw honey

2 Tbsp (30 mL) canola oil

1 Tbsp (15 mL) flaxseed oil

6 cups (1.5 L) watercress (thin stems and leaves only)

1 ripe avocado

For dressing, combine vinegar, onion, apple, soy sauce and honey in a small bowl. Stir in oils. Dressing can be stored covered in refrigerator for up to 2 days; stir or shake well before serving.

Just before serving, place watercress in a large bowl. Drizzle with dressing and toss to coat. Pit and peel avocado, then cut into quarters and slice crosswise into ¼ in (0.5 cm) thick pieces. Add to watercress and toss gently.

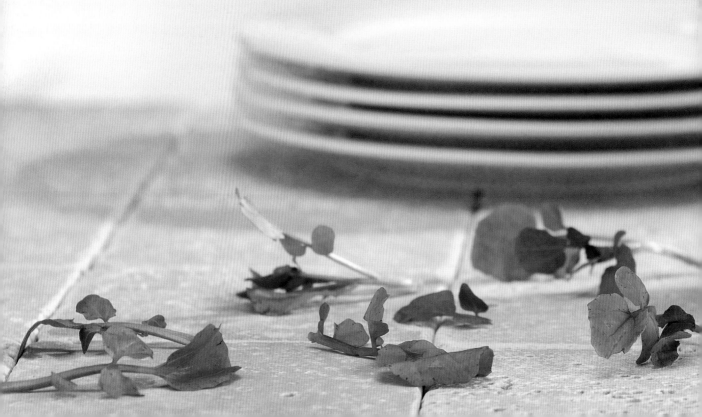

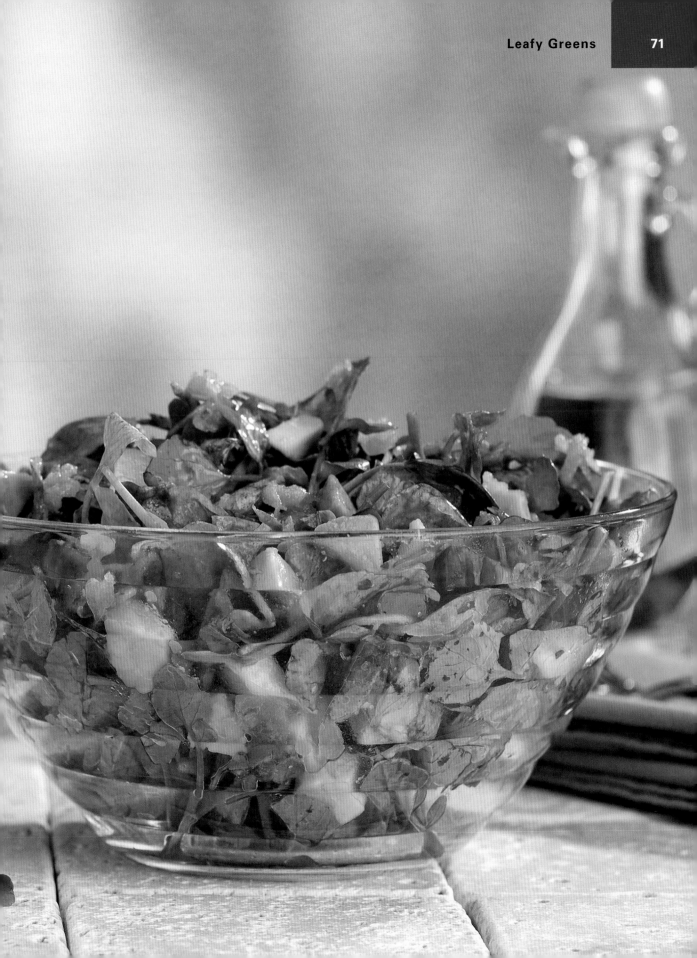

ALL IN THE CABBAGE FAMILY

The Caviar of Irish Food

Cabbage soup, boiled cabbage, and corned beef and cabbage are all dishes that are associated with the Irish, particularly when they receive annual attention in March as individuals worldwide celebrate St. Patrick's Day. Cabbage thrived once it reached the cool climate of the isles and quickly became an important food crop throughout all of Ireland. In the centuries before the potato was introduced, few vegetables could withstand bad weather, so greens such as cabbage and kale, along with leeks and onions, were the main sources of food in winter. By the 1800s, cabbage cultivation allowed for an annual intake of 65 lbs (29 kg) per person per year. During the Irish famine when potato crops began to fail, the Irish relied on cabbage to help them survive. Today, the life-saving cabbage is considered by many to be "the caviar of Irish food."

The Many Faces of Brassica

The wild progenitor of the common cabbage has undergone several transformations as farmers throughout the ages selected particular traits in the plant. Cabbage, collards, broccoli, cauliflower, Brussels sprouts, kohlrabi and hundreds of other cultivars (many of which have now disappeared) all belong to only a single species: *Brassica oleacea*. Wild cabbage can still be seen growing along the jagged cliffs and rocky Atlantic coastlines of Britain, southwestern Europe and the Mediterranean. Selective breeding of the leaves led to the head-forming cabbage and the non-head forming kale; selection of the inflorescence lead to broccoli and cauliflower; and selection of the sprout lead to Brussels sprouts. These vegetables are categorized as cruciferous, named after the shape of their four-petalled flowers that form a cross. The diversity of cruciferous vegetables indicates that breeding was an important activity in ancient times. Every cultivar was prized for its culinary and medicinal values. Today, we reap the benefits of our ancestors' efforts when we consider the vegetables' exceptional content of vitamins, minerals and phytochemicals. Indeed, of all the plants that humans are able to eat, members of the cabbage family probably contain the largest variety of compounds that possess anticancer activity.

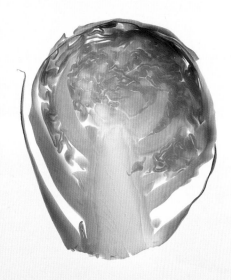

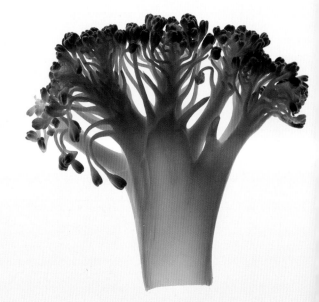

Anticancer Crucifers

Epidemiological research shows that people who eat three or more servings of crucifers per week have a substantially lower risk of developing breast, lung, gastrointestinal, stomach, colorectal and prostate cancers. The compounds that make crucifers such potent anticancer foods are a class of phytochemicals called glucosinolates. These don't act directly to prevent the development of cancer, but instead are broken down by an enzyme, myroinase, that is released from cells of the plant by the action of chewing and digesting. This is where is would be wise to heed your mother's advice to carefully chew your food. The released compounds from glucosinolates can then be classed into isothiocyanates or indoles, both of which possess extremely high anticancer activity. Each crucifer will have a variety of different isothiocyanates and indoles that remain latent in the plant, but that activate when eaten. Broccoli, therefore, has different forms of isothiocyanates and indoles than Brussels sprouts, cabbage and cauliflower.

Crucifers, especially Brussels sprouts, also contain an isothiocyanate called indole-3-carbinol, or I3C, that doesn't contain a sulphur atom and has a different mechanism of action. I3C is able to interfere with estrogen-sensitive tumours such as breast, cervical and uterine cancers. The principal cause of cervical cancer, human papilloma virus HPV16, can be effectively stopped by I3C. It is being tested in phase III clinical trials for the treatment of precancerous cervical dysplasia caused by HPV. In men, I3C is a strong androgen receptor antagonist that is effective against prostate cancer.

To Cook or Not to Cook

The glucosinolates in cruciferous vegetables are soluble in water. To conserve as much of these anticancer compounds as possible, rapid cooking techniques such as steaming or stir-frying in a wok are much preferable to boiling. Myrosinase, the enzyme that breaks down glucosinolate, is also very heat sensitive. To ensure that there's enough of this enzyme to activate isothiocyanates, do not cook your crucifers for too long. The content of both glucosinolates and myrosinases is reduced in frozen vegetables as a result of the blanching process, so try to stick to fresh produce for a vastly superior anticancer superfood. And as a reminder that applies to all of your food, remember to chew carefully.

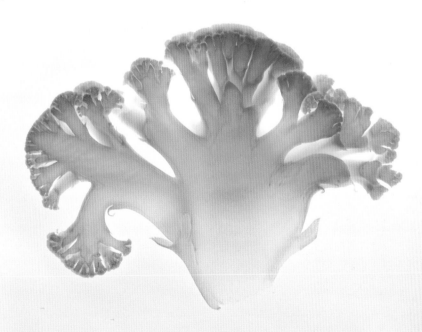

Broccoli

The reputation of broccoli as a health food is well deserved and as a result, consumption has increased 940% over the last 25 years. There is one particular broccoli isothiocyanate that has attracted the attention of researchers as being a powerful anticancer molecule: sulforaphane. Like all isothiocyanates, sulforaphane contains a sulphur atom that is responsible for the characteristic odour released from overcooked crucifers. Research over the last decade indicates that sulforaphane has the ability to flush out toxic substances linked to the development of cancer, causing a significant reduction in the occurrence, number and size of tumours in animals. The molecule appears to work at the site of the tumour itself and induce cellular death (apoptosis). Sulforaphane also acts as a potent antibiotic against *Helicobacter pylori*, the bacteria responsible for stomach ulcers. The presence of ulcers and a *H. pylori* infection is now believed to increase the risk of stomach cancer three- to sixfold. When you eat broccoli, sulforaphane comes in direct contact with *H. pylori* in the stomach and prevents the onset of ulcers.

Lemon Chili Steamed Broccoli

Serves 4

1 bunch of broccoli (about 1³⁄₄ lbs [875 g])

1 tsp (5 mL) canola oil

5 cloves garlic, minced

1 tsp (5 mL) dried crushed chilies

¹⁄₂ cup (125 mL) water

1¹⁄₂ tsp (7 mL) grated lemon zest

³⁄₄ tsp (4 mL) salt

2 cups (500 mL) loosely packed baby arugula leaves

2 Tbsp (30 mL) lemon juice

Trim ¹⁄₂ in (1 cm) from bottom of each broccoli stalk and cut off crowns. Peel stalks and coarsely chop stalks and crowns. Heat oil in a large sauté pan over medium. Add garlic and pepper flakes, and cook, stirring, until fragrant, about 1 to 2 minutes. Add water, broccoli, lemon zest and salt. Cook, stirring, until broccoli is tender-crisp, about 5 minutes. Add arugula and lemon juice. Cook, stirring, until arugula wilts, about 1 minute. Remove from heat and serve immediately.

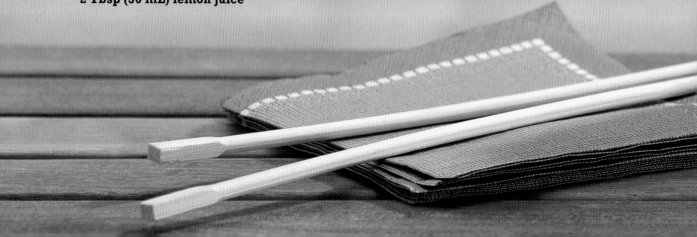

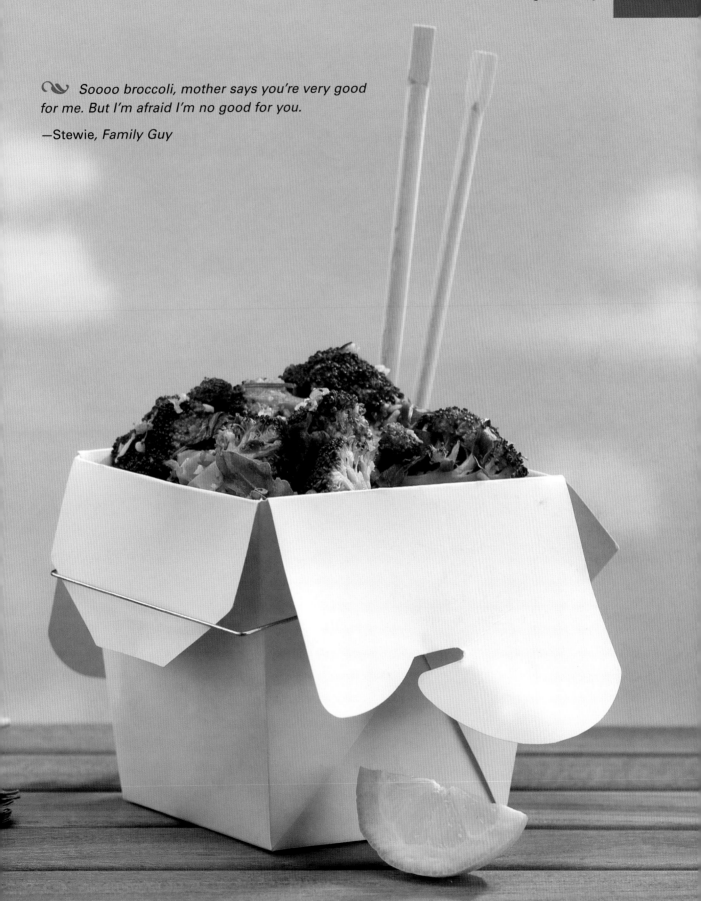

Soooo broccoli, mother says you're very good for me. But I'm afraid I'm no good for you.

—Stewie, *Family Guy*

Roasted Broccoli with Teriyaki Tofu

Serves 4

1 lb (500 g) block extra-firm tofu

2 cups (500 mL) dry sherry

½ cup (125 mL) soy sauce

½ cup (125 mL) water

2 Tbsp (30 mL) minced ginger

2 cloves garlic, minced

2 Tbsp (30 mL) canola oil, *divided*

4 cups (1 L) broccoli florets

Cut tofu blocks in half horizontally to make 2 thick slabs. Lay pieces side by side on a cutting board and place cutting board so that one edge hangs over your sink. Raise other end slightly (even as little as ½ in [1 cm] will be enough so liquid will drain off). Cover with a large plate or second cutting board and lay a heavy weight (such as a phone book or pan of water) on top. Set aside to drain for 30 minutes.

Preheat oven to 400° F (200° C). Combine sherry, soy sauce, water, ginger and garlic in medium sauté pan over medium. Bring to a boil. Cut tofu slabs into 4 triangles each. Add tofu to sauce and simmer for 5 minutes on each side.

Using a slotted spoon, transfer tofu to centre of a lightly oiled, shallow baking dish, reserving sauce. Brush tops and sides lightly with oil (about 2 tsp [10 mL]). Place broccoli in a medium bowl. Drizzle with remaining oil and toss to coat. Add broccoli florets to baking dish around tofu. Pour reserved sauce over top. Bake until broccoli is tender-crisp (it may brown slightly). Serve immediately.

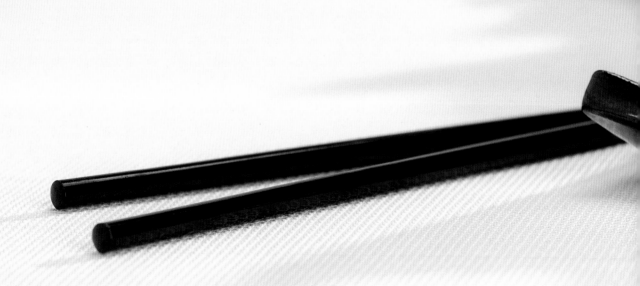

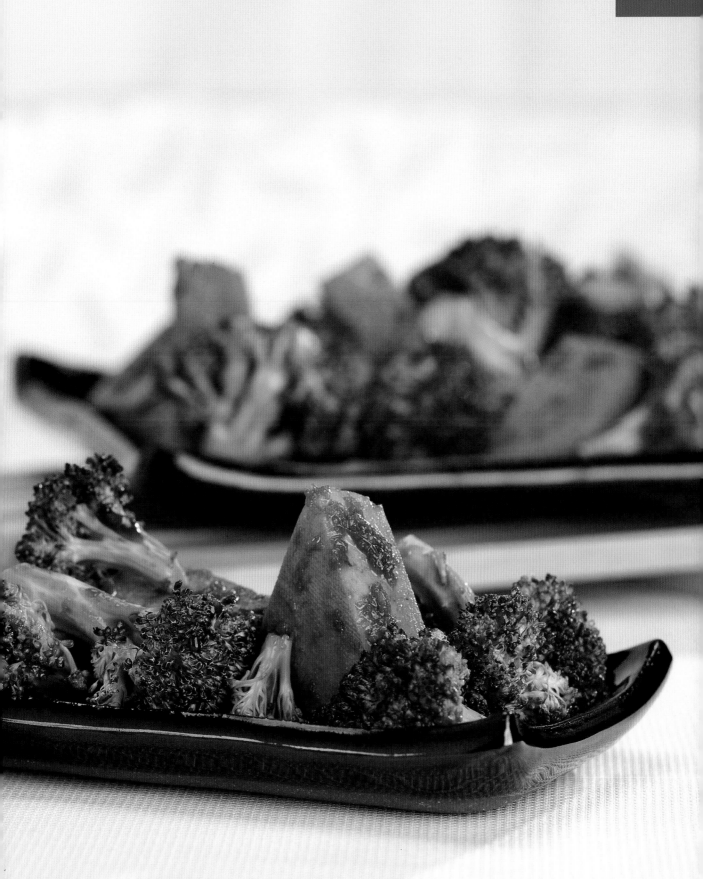

Brussels Sprouts

These smelly little mini cabbages originated in Belgium, where they have been cultivated since the 12th century, and I'm sure many people would be happy to just let them stay there. We've all suffered through mounds of poorly prepared Brussels sprouts, boiled into mush and barely recognizable, which is probably why so many people give an involuntary shudder of revulsion when they think of this super nutritious veggie. Even the fact that the sprouts are loaded with vitamins C and K (you can get your entire daily requirement for both vitamins by eating only 5 sprouts!) isn't enough to tempt some people into adding Brussels sprouts to their menu. Well, these people are missing out. When roasted or stir-fried, Brussels sprouts are delicious, and they pack a nutritional punch. An excellent source of fibre, potassium and glucosinolates, sprouts may help prevent some forms of cancer, such as colon, lung, prostate and breast cancers, and may also protect against rheumatoid arthritis.

Roasted Brussels Sprouts with Hazelnuts and Pomegranate

Serves 4

1 Tbsp (15 mL) grape seed oil

1 Tbsp (15 mL) pomegranate molasses

1 Tbsp (15 mL) chopped fresh oregano

1/8 tsp (0.5 mL) each salt and freshly ground pepper

1 lb (500 g) Brussels sprouts, trimmed and cut in half lengthwise

2 Tbsp (30 mL) pomegranate seeds

2 Tbsp (30 mL) toasted sliced hazelnuts

For marinade, combine oil, pomegranate molasses, oregano, salt and pepper in small bowl. Mix well. Place Brussels sprouts in a large bowl. Drizzle with marinade and toss to coat. Chill for 30 minutes.

Preheat oven to 350° F (175° C). Arrange sprouts, cut side down, in a large shallow baking pan. Roast, without turning, until tender, about 45 minutes. Toss with pomegranate seeds and hazelnuts. Transfer to a serving dish.

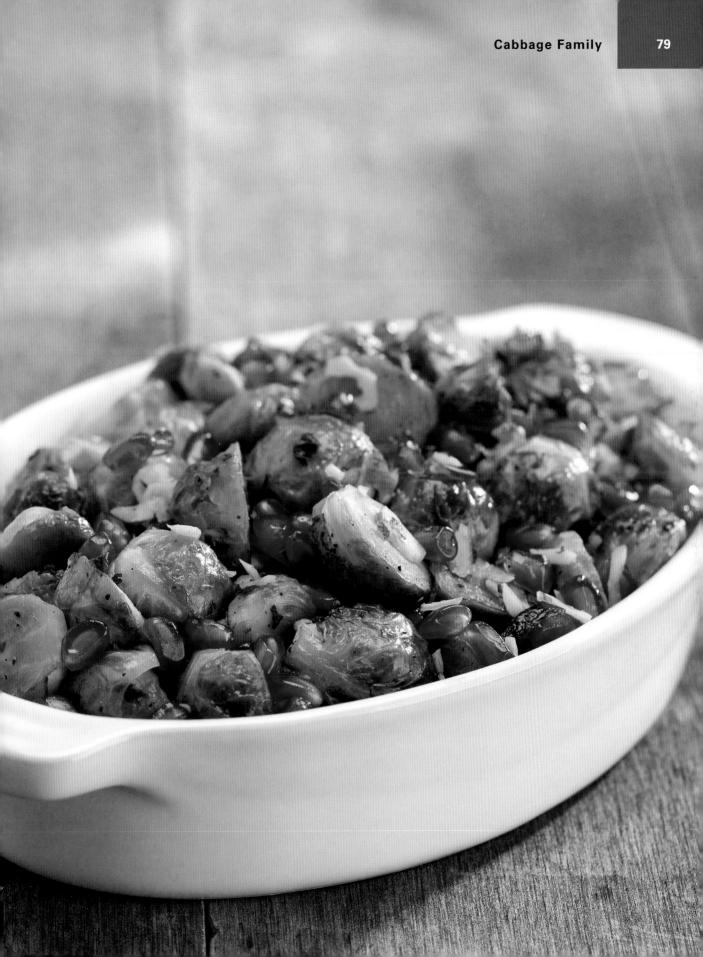

Spiced Slivered Brussels Sprouts with Orange

Serves 4

1 lb (500 g) Brussels sprouts

⅔ cup (160 mL) freshly squeezed orange juice

2 Tbsp (30 mL) lemon juice

2 tsp (10 mL) raw honey

¼ tsp (1 mL) sea salt

½ tsp (2 mL) cayenne pepper

1 tsp (5 mL) caraway seeds

1 Tbsp (15 mL) canola oil

2 tsp (10 mL) orange zest

4 green onions, thinly sliced, keeping light and dark parts separate

Trim Brussels sprouts stem ends flush. Cut vertically into ½ in (1 cm) thick slices. Transfer to a medium bowl and add lukewarm water to cover. Top with a plate to keep Brussels sprouts submerged.

Combine orange and lemon juices, honey, sea salt and cayenne in a small bowl. Stir until honey has dissolved.

Heat caraway seeds in a large, dry sauté pan over medium. Cook, stirring constantly, until fragrant and starting to pop, about 2 to 3 minutes. Transfer seeds to cutting board and chop. Heat oil in same sauté pan over medium. Add orange zest and light parts of green onion. Cook, stirring, until fragrant, about 1 minute. Add Brussels sprouts slices and increase heat to high. Cook, stirring, until wilted, about 2 minutes. Add juice mixture and reduce heat to medium-high. Cook, stirring, until juice has evaporated, about 4 minutes. Stir in dark parts of green onions and caraway seeds. Serve immediately.

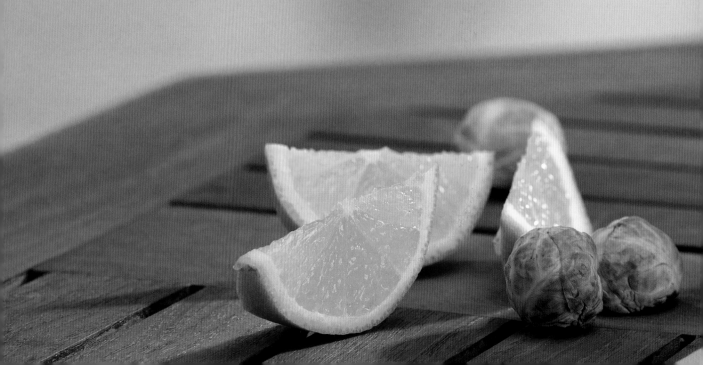

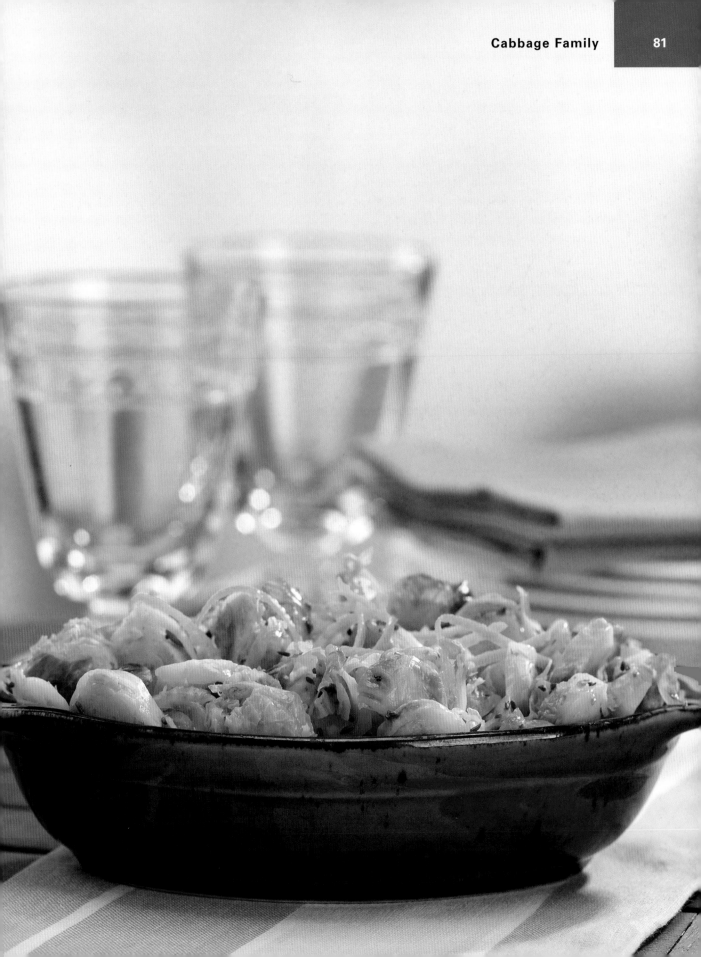

Cabbage

Not only is there a wide diversity of plants within the cabbage family, there are also many different varieties of cabbage itself—green, red, Savoy (or curly) and Napa (which deviates in appearance from the head cabbages and looks a lot like romaine lettuce) are some of the most common. All varieties of cabbage are loaded with polyphenols, antioxidants that help prevent oxidative stress and are known for their anticancer activity; red cabbage is particularly high in anthocyanins, which are among the most powerful antioxidants and have anti-inflamatory properties. The glucosinolates found in cabbage help protect against bladder, breast, colon and prostate cancer, and are also known to protect the digestive tract and the stomach lining, helping reduce the risk of ulcers. As for vitamins, cabbage is an excellent source of vitamin C and K, and a good source of vitamin A and folate.

Grilled Tofu and Cabbage Salad

Serves 4

3 Tbsp (45 mL) rice vinegar

6 Tbsp (90 mL) soy sauce, *divided*

1 Tbsp (15 mL) agave nectar or raw honey

¼ tsp (1 mL) sesame oil

¼ tsp (1 mL) Sriracha sauce

¾ cup (175 mL) julienned grilled tofu (see p. 100)

2 cups (500 mL) shredded green cabbage

1½ cups (375 mL) shredded red cabbage

½ cup (125 mL) julienned carrot

Combine rice vinegar, soy sauce, agave nectar, sesame oil and Sriracha sauce in a small bowl. Whisk well to combine.

Combine tofu, cabbages and carrot in a large bowl. Drizzle with dressing and toss to coat. Cover and refrigerate for at least 30 minutes before serving.

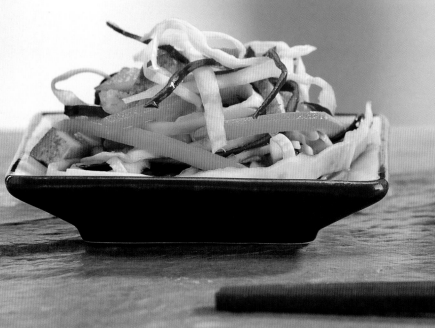

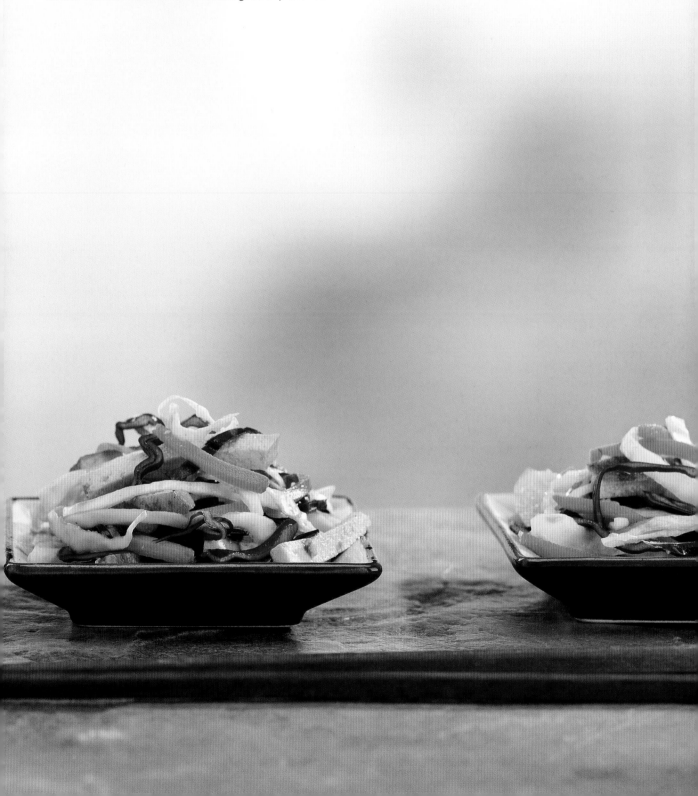

Sriracha is a Thai hot chili pepper paste available in the Asian food aisle of most grocery stores.

Cabbage Kimchi

Makes 8 cups (2 L)

1 to 2 large Napa cabbages
(about 4 lbs [1.8 kg])

1 large daikon radish
(1½ to 2 lbs [750 to 1000 g]),
julienned into 2 in (5 cm)
long pieces

5 Tbsp (75 mL) coarse sea
salt

1 cup (250 mL) filtered
water

⅓ cup (80 mL) unseasoned
rice vinegar

1½ Tbsp (22 mL) rice flour

¼ cup (60 mL) Korean fine
or medium ground red chili
powder (see Tip)

6 cloves garlic, minced

2 Tbsp (30 mL) minced
ginger

2 Tbsp (30 mL) Korean red
chili flakes (see Tip)

1 bunch of watercress,
tough stems trimmed

3 green onions, julienned
into 2 in (5 cm) long pieces

Make sure all work surfaces, vessels and utensils are
spotlessly clean before beginning. Trim and discard tough
outer leaves of cabbage. Cut cabbage in half lengthwise,
and trim and discard core. Cut cabbage crosswise in 2 in
(5 cm) wide strips. Place strips in a large bowl, add daikon
and salt, and toss to combine. Transfer to a colander. Place
a plate on colander and top with a weight, such as a
saucepan full of water. Set aside for 24 hours.

Combine filtered water with rice vinegar in a small
saucepan. Bring to a boil over high heat; remove from heat
and set aside to cool completely. Transfer to a large bowl.
Stir in rice flour, chili powder, garlic, ginger and chili flakes
until well combined. Add watercress and green onion and
stir to combine. Working in batches, place cabbage and
daikon mixture in a kitchen towel and twist to wring out
excess moisture, then add to mixture in bowl. Once all
cabbage mixture has been added, toss to coat well. Pack
into two 1 quart (4 cup [1 L]) sterilized glass jars. Screw lids
on tightly. Let stand at room temperature for 48 hours,
then transfer to refrigerator to chill for 4 days before eating.
Eat within 3 weeks. Shown served with a Korean dish
called Bi Bim Baap.

Tip

Do not substitute regular chili powder or pepper flakes for
the Korean versions called for in the recipe, as they are
quite different.

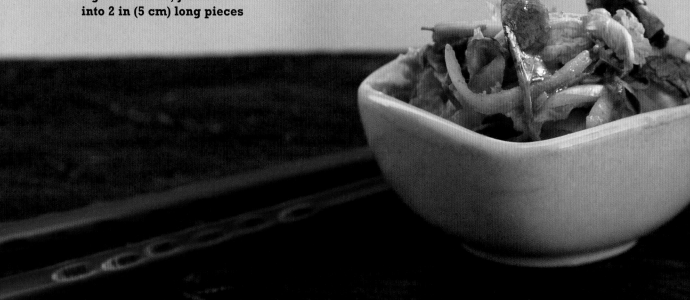

The Romans and Greeks prized cabbage as an important medicinal plant. Cato the Elder (234–149 BC), a powerful Roman statesman, was the first to use the term brassica, from the Celtic bresic, or "cabbage." Mistrustful of physicians, who all happened to be Greek at the time, Cato believed cabbage to be a universal cure-all with life-preserving properties. In his agricultural treatise De Agri Cultura ("On Farming") he provides the prototype for coleslaw: "..eaten raw with vinegar, or cooked in oil or other fat, cabbage gets rid of all and heals all."

However, not all of his recommendations sound as appealing. In the same book, he suggests to "...store the urine of anyone who habitually eats cabbage; warm it, bathe the patient in it. With this treatment you will soon restore health; it has been tested...Those who cannot see clearly should bathe their eyes in this urine and they will see more." Cato fathered a child at 80 years old and he attributes his virility to cabbage, so consider his advice wisely.

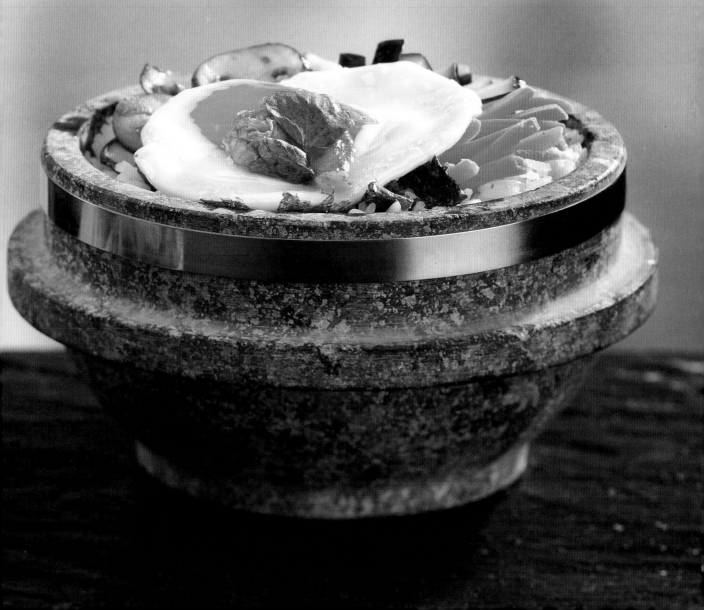

Cauliflower

The name "cauliflower" comes from *caulis,* the Latin word for cabbage, clearly stating this vegetables place in the cabbage family. In fact, members of the cabbage family are so closely related that until about 60 years ago, broccoli was considered a type of cauliflower. Although the white variety is the most common, cauliflower also has orange, green and purple varieties, all of which are high in fibre, folate and calcium and are significant sources of omega-3 fatty acids. Cauliflower is also a good source of indoles—phytochemicals that help protect against skin, breast and prostate cancers. And like the rest of the crucifers, cauliflower contains sulforaphane, known for its anticancer activity.

Creamy Golden Cauliflower Soup

Serves 6

2 medium heads of cauliflower, cut into 1 in (2.5 cm) pieces

2³⁄₄ cups (675 mL) milk, *divided*

2³⁄₄ cups (675 mL) vegetable stock, *divided*

1 Tbsp (15 mL) turmeric

salt and white pepper to taste

Place cauliflower, 2 cups (500 mL) of milk, 2 cups (500 mL) of vegetable stock and turmeric in a large saucepan. Bring to a boil over medium high, then reduce heat to low and cook until cauliflower is very tender, about 20 minutes. Purée with a hand blender, or in batches in a blender, until smooth. Return to low heat and stir in remaining ³⁄₄ cup (80 mL) each of milk and stock. Stir in salt and white pepper. Heat until warmed through, then serve immediately.

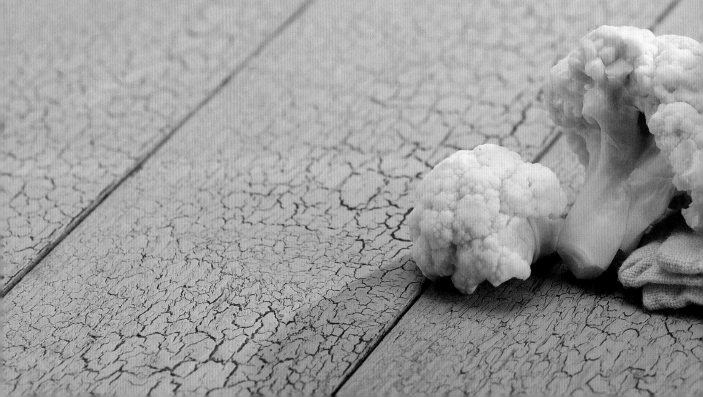

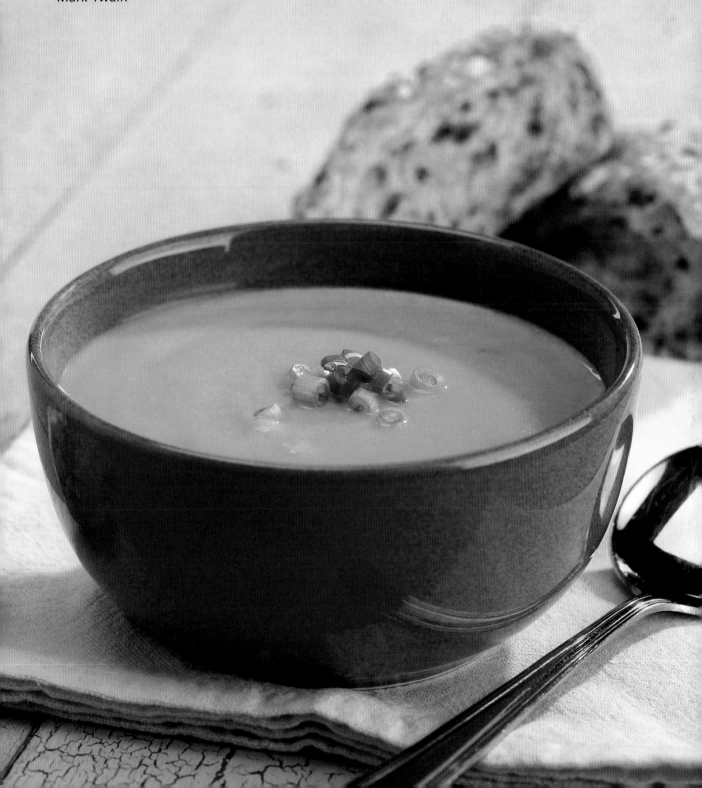

Cauliflower is nothing but cabbage with a college education.

—Mark Twain

Baked Cauliflower in Tomato Sauce

Serves 6

1 Tbsp (15 mL) whole coriander seeds

1½ tsp (7 mL) whole cumin seeds

½ tsp (2 mL) fennel seeds

1 Tbsp (15 mL) canola oil

1 medium onion, finely chopped

1 clove garlic, minced

1½ Tbsp (22 mL) minced ginger

½ tsp (2 mL) turmeric

½ tsp (2 mL) cayenne

¾ tsp (4 mL) sea salt

1 tsp (5 mL) agave nectar

1½ cups (375 mL) tomato juice

1 medium head of cauliflower, leaves cut off

½ cup (125 mL) chopped fresh cilantro

⅓ cup (80 mL) chopped macadamia nuts

plain fat-free yogurt, optional

Preheat oven to 350° F (175° C). Combine coriander, cumin and fennel seeds in a small dry sauté pan over medium heat. Toast, stirring, until fragrant, about 1 to 2 minutes. Transfer to a spice mill or mortar and grind to a fine powder.

Heat oil in a medium sauté pan over medium. Add onion and garlic and cook, stirring, until softened, about 3 minutes. Add ginger, turmeric, cayenne, salt and toasted spice mixture. Cook, stirring, for another minute. Stir in agave. Add tomato juice and bring to a boil, stirring occasionally. Cover, reduce heat to low and simmer for 5 minutes.

Rinse cauliflower. Trim ½ in (1 cm) from bottom of stalk. Remove florets and cut into small pieces, leaving as little stem attached as possible. Peel thick part of stem and chop into small pieces, keeping separate from florets. Spread stem pieces in a shallow 7 x 11 in (18 x 28 cm) baking dish. Spread florets on top, then spoon sauce over. Cover and bake until tender, about 30 to 35 minutes. Remove cover and continue to bake until liquid has evaporated and top has browned, about 10 to 15 minutes more.

To serve, sprinkle with cilantro and macadamia nuts, and top individual portions with a dollop of yogurt, if desired.

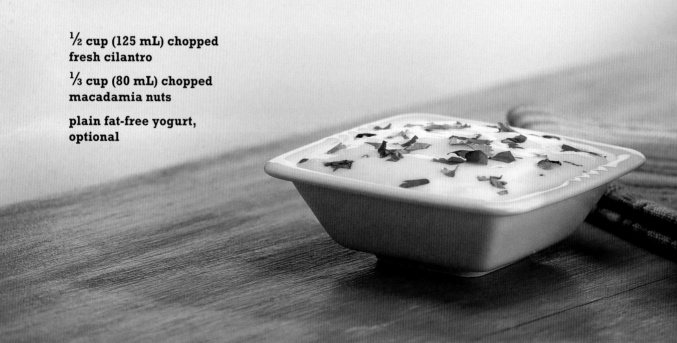

A staple in Indian cuisine, turmeric has a distinctive golden hue—which seems only fitting when you consider how valuable this spice is for our health. Turmeric has anti-inflammatory properties that are as effective as some anti-inflammatory medications (including phenylbutazone) but do not have the negative side effects; it has traditionally been used to treat arthritis. Turmeric also has anticancer properties, improves liver function and may help protect against cystic fibrosis and neurodegenerative diseases such as Alzheimer's.

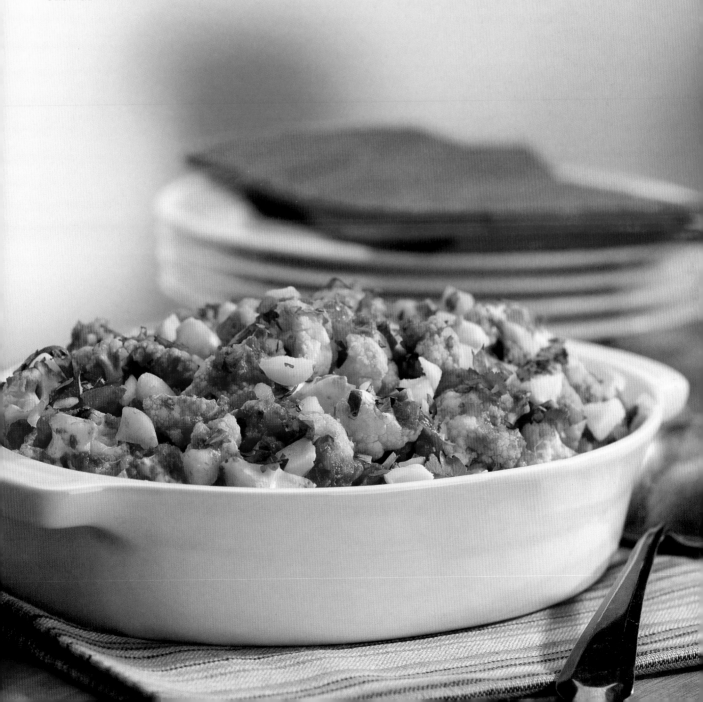

Don't Spill the Beans

A Hill of Beans

A single species, *Phaseolus vulgaris* or the common bean, is responsible for at least 500 varieties of bean, including green, black, red, white, yellow, kidney, lima, mung, navy, pinto and string beans. All varieties of *P. vulgaris* originated in Peru, where seeds that date back more than 7000 years have been discovered in deposits in Guitarrero Cave in the Callejon de Huaylas. Similar deposits have also been discovered in Tehuacán, Mexico. To Native Americans, beans, along with corn and squash, comprised the Three Sisters. The crops were grown with a method of companion plant cultivation in which corn acted as a trellis for the beans and provided shade for squash; beans fixed the nitrogen for corn and squash; and squash detered herbivores because of its coarse, hairy leaves. The crops also complemented each other nutritionally in that beans supplied an amino acid that was missing in corn and vice-versa, providing a complete protein profile. Christopher Columbus introduced the common bean to Europe in 1493 when he returned from his second voyage to the New World. The bean spread to the eastern Mediterranean and by the 1600s was cultivated everywhere in Italy, Greece and Turkey. Beans of the *Phaseolus* genus were a new addition to those that originated in the Old World, such as broad beans (genus *Vicia*), chickpeas (genus *Cicer*), peas (genus *Pisum*), lentils (genus *Lens*) and soy (genus *Glycine*).

Small but Mighty

Beans and lentils are one of the best (and least expensive) sources of dietary fibre, which helps stabilize blood sugar levels—a necessary step in preventing or treating insulin resistance, hyperglycemia and type 2 diabetes. Another healthy consequence of fibre is its cholesterol-reducing ability. A study that followed close to 10,000 American adults for 19 years showed that those who ate the most high-fibre foods such as beans or lentils had 12% less heart disease and 11% less cardiovascular disease than those who ate less. Beans and lentils also contain phytochemicals such as diosgenin, protease inhibitors and phytic acid, all of which have anticancer properties. And as any vegetarian knows, legumes are good sources of protein, which is essential for building and repairing tissue in the body.

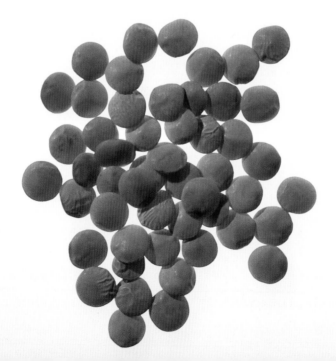

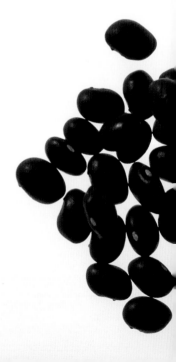

The Toot and Nothing but the Toot

The bean owes its musical prowess to short-chain sugars, particularly raffinose and stachyose, which require an enzyme that humans do not produce. Consequently, they pass right thought the small intestine unscathed and end up being digested by bacteria residing in the colon. The bacteria produce flatulence-causing gases as a byproduct. To reduce any embarrassing musical talent, soak the beans for several hours in water before cooking them. Some spices, such as anise seeds, coriander and cumin, can act as carminatives (substances that relieve flatulence) and be added to bean dishes.

It's Bean Nice Knowing You...

In most societies, the bean has been associated with birth or death. The ancient Egyptians believed that the souls of the newly dead awaited reincarnation in a place called "the beanfield." To the ancient Greeks and Romans, beans symbolized the dead, and to some, they literally contained the souls of the dead. We may remember Pythagoras from our trigonometry classes, but he also founded a religion that touted vegetarianism, reincarnation, sexual equity and the well-tempered musical scale. Among his taboos, the worst was to eat beans. This drastic statement is based on the theory from one of his peers, Diogenes Laertius, who stated that beans are "the material which contain the largest portion of that animal matter which our souls are made of." The Greek word for soul was *anemos*, which also meant wind, and it was believed that buried people released their souls in the form of wind or gas, which was then absorbed into the beans. When you ate beans, the passing gas was the escaped souls of the dead who would then ascend to heaven. To Pythagoras, eating beans denoted devouring one's own parents, and thus causing a major upset in the reincarnation cycle. So strong were his convictions that he refused to escape his murderers by crossing a beanfield.

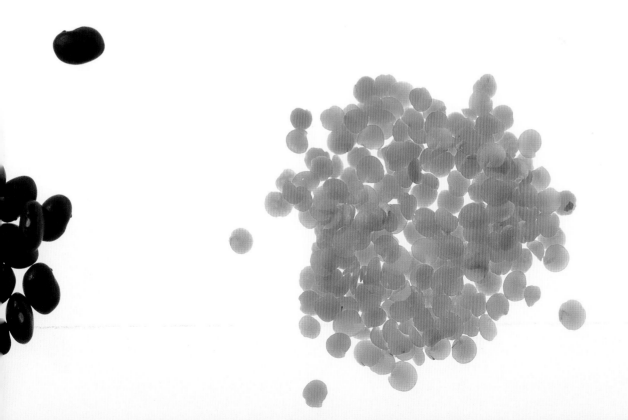

Black Beans

Not only are black beans an excellent source of protein and fibre (15 g per cup for both), they are also rich in flavonoids. Researchers have discovered eight different types of flavonoids—including anthocyanins, which are generally associated with berries or red wine—in the beans' seat coat. These powerful antioxidants help protect against cardiovascular disease and have anti-inflammatory properties. Black beans also help keep the digestive tract healthy; they allow bacteria in the digestive tract to produce butyric acid, which has anti-inflammatory effects and helps protect against colon cancer. And although they may not be on par with fish as a source of omega-3 fatty acids, black beans contain about three times the amount of omega-3s found in other legumes.

Black Bean Hummus

Makes about 3 cups (750 mL)

1 cup (250 mL) dried black beans

3 cups (750 mL) cold water

¼ cup (60 mL) tahini

5 Tbsp (75 mL) lime juice

2 Tbsp (30 mL) olive oil

3 cloves garlic, minced

2 tsp (10 mL) ground cumin

1 tsp (5 mL) cayenne pepper

salt and pepper to taste

¼ cup (60 mL) packed chopped fresh cilantro

At room temperature, soak beans in water to cover for at least 4 hours and up to overnight. Drain and place in a medium saucepan with 3 cups (750 mL) cold water. Bring to a boil over medium-high. Reduce heat, cover partially and simmer until beans are tender, about 1½ hours. Drain and cool to room temperature before continuing.

Combine beans, tahini, lime juice, oil, garlic, cumin and cayenne in food processor. Process until smooth. Add salt and pepper to taste. Add cilantro and pulse with an on/off motion until cilantro is incorporated. Serve with fresh vegetables for dipping or use as a sandwich spread. Keep covered in refrigerator for up to 5 days.

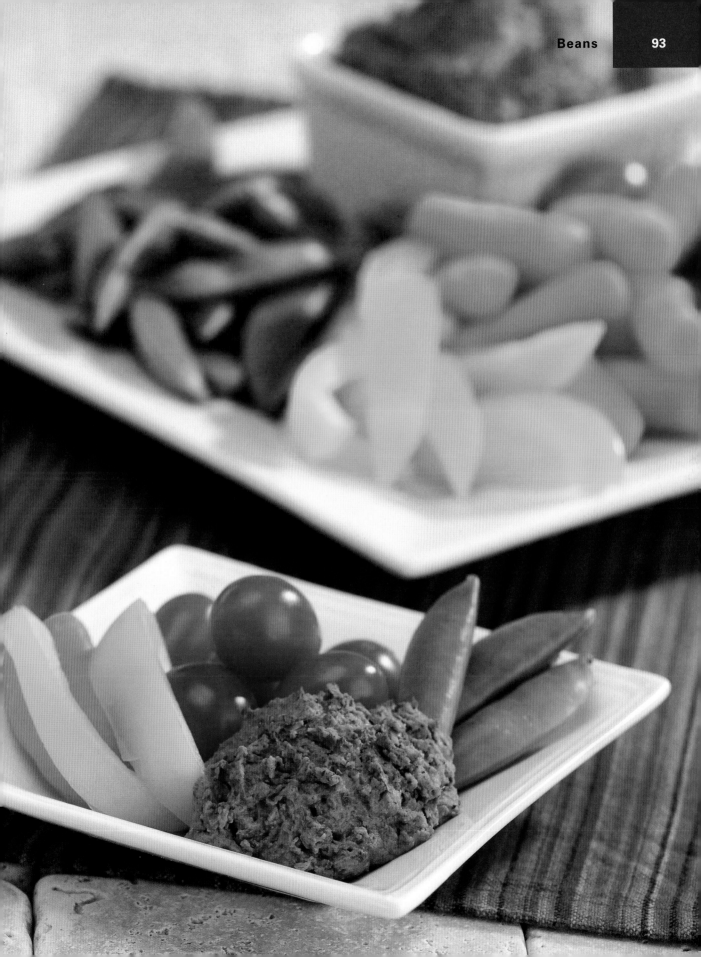

Lentils

Lentils range in colour from yellow to red to deep black, and all of them provide twice as much iron as other legumes. They are rich in both types of dietary fibres, soluble and insoluble, which not only help to increase stool bulk and decrease constipation, but also lower cholesterol and prevent gastrointestinal disorders such as diverticulosis and irritable bowel syndrome. Lentils' contribution to heart health is also boosted by their significant amounts of folate and magnesium. Folate is necessary to lower blood levels of homocysteine, an intermediate product in the methylation cycle that can directly damage artery walls. Magnesium plays an important role in regulating blood pressure and is considered essential for those suffering from hypertension.

French Lentils with Mint and Sorrel

Serves 6

1 cup (250 mL) French lentils

3 cups (750 mL) cold water

2¾ tsp (14 mL) salt, *divided*

2 Tbsp (30 mL) canola oil

1 clove garlic, minced

1 Tbsp (15 mL) minced ginger

½ cup (125 mL) finely chopped carrots

1 cup (250 mL) unsweetened apple juice

3 Tbsp (45 mL) apple cider vinegar

¼ cup (125 mL) finely chopped fresh mint

¼ cup finely chopped sorrel

pepper

¼ cup (60 mL) mint chiffonade

Rinse lentils well in cold water and check carefully for any small stones. Bring at least 3 cups (750 mL) water to a boil in a medium saucepan with 2 tsp (10 mL) salt. Add lentils and boil until *al dente*, about 20 minutes. Drain. (Lentils can be prepared ahead up to this point, then refreshed under cold running water and refrigerated until needed.)

Heat oil in a large sauté pan over medium. Add garlic, ginger and carrots, and cook, stirring, until fragrant, about 1 to 2 minutes. Add lentils, apple juice and ¾ tsp (4 mL) salt. Cook, stirring occasionally, until liquid has absorbed, about 10 minutes. Add vinegar, mint and sorrel. Season to taste with pepper. Transfer to a serving dish. Sprinkle mint chiffonade overtop.

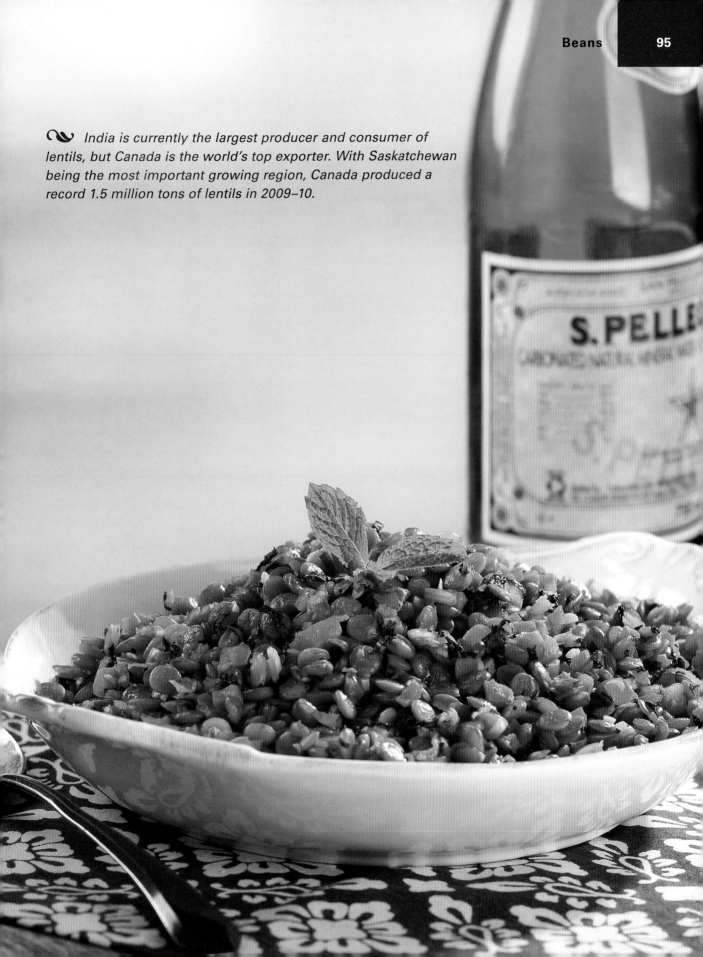

India is currently the largest producer and consumer of lentils, but Canada is the world's top exporter. With Saskatchewan being the most important growing region, Canada produced a record 1.5 million tons of lentils in 2009–10.

Soy: The Most Widely Eaten Plant on the Planet

Soy Many Choices...

From tofu and burgers to ice cream and baby formula, soy products have been heralded as a healthy source of quality protein with a reputation for being all natural and all good. They've become the almost ideal substitute for animal proteins, welcomed by vegetarians and those who shun dietary cholesterol and saturated fats. As the evidence of soy's health benefits kept accumulating, sales and consumption skyrocketed. From 1996 to 2009, soy food sales increased from $300 million to nearly $4.5 billion, and between 2000 and 2007, more than 2700 new soy-based foods and products were introduced by U.S. food manufacturers. Walk into any grocery store in North America today and you'll be sure to find a huge variety of soy stuff.

Isoflavones Hold Their Own

The popularity of soy really took off as a health food in the early 1900s after nutrition pioneer George Washington Carver and breakfast cereal inventor John Harvey Kellogg began promoting the "greater bean's" health benefits. Soy is an excellent source of protein and provides essential fatty acids, numerous vitamins and minerals, dietary fibre, and isoflavones, the bean's principal phytochemical compound. Isoflavones have been extensively studied for their capacity to influence a number of events associated with the uncontrolled growth of cancer cells.

The major isoflavones in soybeans are genistein and daidzen, classified as phytoestrogens because of their resemblance, at the molecular level, to estrogens. Isoflavones are thought to act as anti-estrogens because they can bind to estrogen receptor sites. Estrogen is a powerful stimulator of cell growth, and chronically high levels in the blood may trigger uncontrolled cell growth leading to cancer. Hormone-dependent cancers such as breast and prostate cancers, the primary causes of cancer deaths in North America, can be positively affected if phytoestrogens block estrogen's biological effects. Indeed, numerous epidemiological studies suggest that the low incidence of these cancers in Asian populations is a result of the frequent consumption of soy. Japanese women who had the most consistently high levels of genistein had the lowest rates of breast cancer.

Paradoxically, this association was not observed in North America. Among all the factors offered by researchers to explain why soy is healthy in the East, but not in the West, the most important one concerns the source of isoflavones and the type of soy consumed. This is further complicated by several population and laboratory studies that suggest that isoflavones only prevent breast cancer if consumed before or during puberty, as it affects how breast tissue develops. Women who begin consuming soy later in life may not see any benefit.

East vs. West

Experts believe that the principal reason behind soy's controversial status as a health food or as a health risk lies in the type and quantity of soy consumed. In Asia, the intake of traditional soy-based foods is relatively high, with fermented soy foods such as miso and natto accounting for 40%. In the West, consumption of traditional soy foods is much lower. Instead, isoflavones are consumed from the plethora of non-soy based foods that have added soy protein and flour. Interestingly, doughnuts provided 20% of soy isoflavones in a sample of 447 women living in San Francisco. Virtually every processed or manufactured food contains some soy ingredient, from textured vegetable protein to the generic ingredient "vegetable oil." Soy oil is the most widely

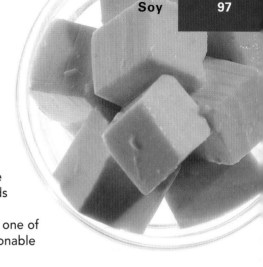

used oil in the U.S. and Canada, accounting for more than 75% of our total vegetable fats and oil intake, most of it hydrogenated. It is the most widely eaten plant in the world, and never in human history has this much "hidden" soy been consumed. How this will affect long-term public health is unknown, but critics caution that such an experiment should not be conducted without careful monitoring and vigilance.

An additional concern is the fact that 93% of the U.S. and 60% of the Canadian soybean crop is genetically engineered. More than two-thirds of transgenic soy is genetically altered to withstand glyphosate-containing herbicides. Consequently, soybeans in North America are one of the most highly sprayed crops and contain residues that have questionable health effects.

The Heart Truth

In 1999, the evidence for the heart-protective effects of soy was convincing enough that the U.S. Food and Drug Administration approved labelling for foods containing soy protein with the following health claim "25 grams/day of soy protein, as part of a diet low in saturated fat and cholesterol, may reduce the risk of heart disease." An American Heart Association review of a decade-long study on soy protein's cardiovascular benefits concluded that soy protein does lower LDL cholesterol, but the effect is a modest 3%, and only if soy protein intake is extremely high (more than 50% of daily protein intake). No benefit was evident on HDL cholesterol, triglycerides, lipoprotein(a) or blood pressure. Health Canada's Food Directorate came to their own conclusion that "overall, existing data are inconsistent or inadequate in supporting most of the suggested health benefits of consuming soy protein or isoflavones." Nevertheless, soy products in Canada do contain health claims regarding postmenopausal symptoms and bone mineral density loss, based on a number of small studies that showed attenuation or improvement. A recent well-designed study however found no effect, prompting the *Time* magazine headline "Hot Flash Flop: Soy does nothing to ease symptoms of menopause."

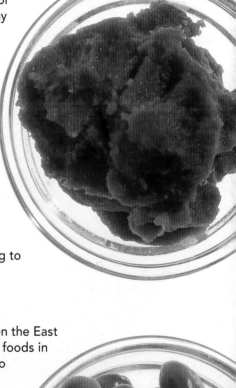

Good Soy, Bad Soy

The great differences in the rates of hormone-dependent cancers between the East and West can be attributable to the consumption of traditional soy-based foods in Asian countries, especially if consumption begins before puberty. If you do decide to make soy part of your diet, ensure that it is in the whole and/or fermented form. The highly processed, highly sprayed, highly genetically modified and highly marketed soy that is eaten in North America (classified not as a legume, but as an oilseed by the Food and Agriculture Organization [FAO]) bears little resemblance to the original *Glycine max* native to East Asia. Soy can indeed be considered a powerful superfood, but the term needs to be narrowed considerably to include only a very small segment of all the soy products and forms available today. Soy many products, soy little choice...

Miso

Soybeans made their way into Chinese kitchens sometime after the Zhou Dynasty (1122–256 BC), but only in their fermented forms, such as miso and soy sauce. Miso and other fermented soy products are some of the richest sources of vitamin K2 (menatetrenon, MK4), an essential nutrient involved in maintaining bone mineral density, enhancing memory and preventing vascular damage. Miso is also a good source of zinc, which helps strengthen the immune system. Natto, another popular fermented form of soy, contains nattokinase, an enzyme that has potent fibrinolytic activity able to break blood clots and thus reduce the risk of thrombosis.

Cabbage and Miso Soup

Serves 4

3 cups (750 mL) vegetable stock

2 cups (500 mL) chopped green cabbage

1 cup (250 mL) sweet potato cut in ½ in (1 cm) cubes

1 stalk of celery, sliced diagonally ¼ in (0.5 cm) thick

½ carrot, thinly sliced

4 cloves garlic, minced

1 Tbsp (15 mL) minced ginger

3 green onions, thinly sliced

2 Tbsp (30 mL) plus 2 tsp (10 mL) red miso

a few drops of sesame oil, to taste

Bring stock to a boil in a medium saucepan. Add cabbage, sweet potato, celery, carrot, garlic and ginger. Cover, reduce heat to medium-low and simmer until vegetables are tender, about 10 minutes. Stir in green onion and turn off heat. Measure miso into a small bowl. Add a ladleful of soup broth and stir until miso has dissolved. Pour back into saucepan and stir. To serve, ladle into bowls and add a few drops of sesame oil to each bowl.

Soy cultivation originated in China over 13,000 years ago. But before it became an important food crop, it was used in crop rotation as a method of fixing nitrogen to fertilize the soil for other food crops.

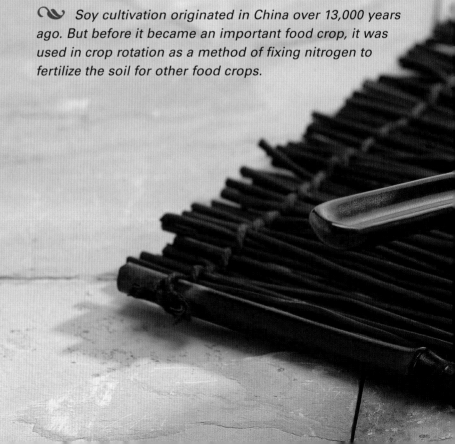

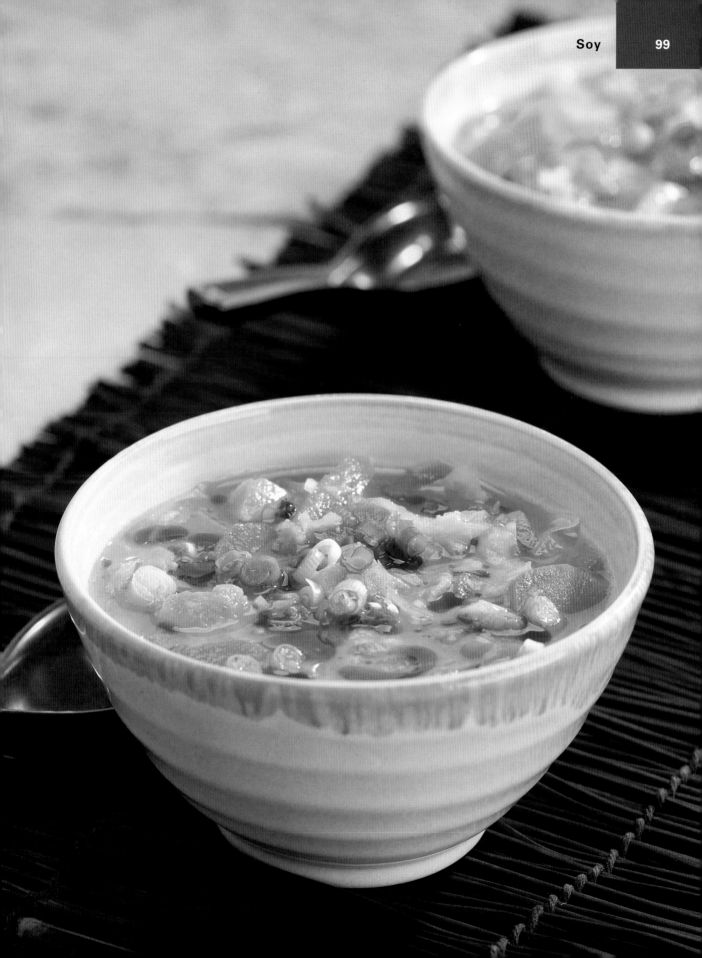

Tofu

Tofu originated in the Han Dynasty, and it involved the pulverization of soybeans that had been previously soaked in water, leading to the extraction of a whitish liquid, or "milk" that was then coagulated with minerals, mild acids or salts. Although tofu itself doesn't have much flavour, it is prized for its versatility in that it takes on the flavours of the ingredients it is cooked with. Tofu also boasts a high protein content and is a good source of iron, copper, manganese and Omega-3 fatty acids.

Marinated Grilled Tofu

Serves 4

2 x 1 lb (500 g) blocks extra-firm tofu

4 tsp (20 mL) canola oil, divided

4 tsp (20 mL) tamari

2 Tbsp (30 mL) rice vinegar

2 tsp (10 mL) sesame oil

2 cloves garlic, minced

1 green onion, thinly sliced

¼ cup (60 mL) hoisin sauce

2 Tbsp (30 mL) balsamic vinegar

1 Tbsp (15 mL) minced ginger

1 Tbsp (15 mL) orange juice

½ tsp (2 mL) toasted sesame seeds, optional

Cut blocks of tofu in half horizontally to make 2 thick slabs from each block. Arrange on a cutting board and place board so that one edge hangs over your sink. Raise other end slightly (even as little as ½ in [1 cm] is enough) so liquid will drain off. Cover with a large plate or second cutting board and lay a heavy weight (such as a phone book or a pan of water) on top. Set aside to drain for 30 minutes. Heat 1 tsp (5 mL) of canola oil in a large sauté pan over medium-high. Add tofu and cook until golden brown on bottom, about 5 minutes. Flip and cook until golden on second side, another 5 minutes.

Combine tamari, rice vinegar, sesame oil, garlic and green onion in a shallow dish. Add tofu, turning to coat all sides with marinade. Cover and refrigerate for at least 2 hours and up to 2 days, turning occasionally.

Preheat grill to medium high. Remove tofu from refrigerator 30 minutes before grilling. Stir together hoisin, balsamic vinegar, ginger and orange juice in a small bowl. Drain tofu and discard marinade. Rub with remaining canola oil. Place on preheated greased grill and cook about 5 minutes per side, brushing occasionally with hoisin mixture.

To serve, cut each piece into 2 triangles and sprinkle with sesame seeds.

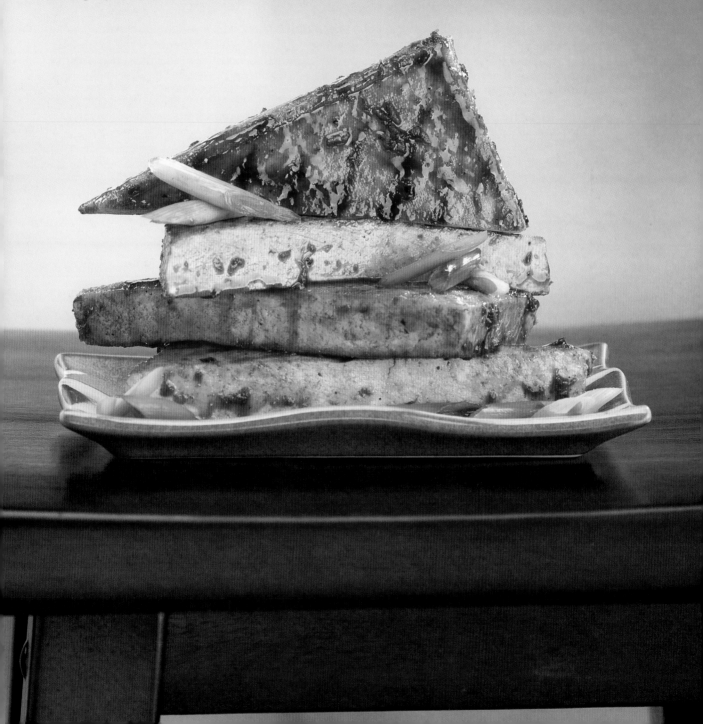 Soy milk, contrary to popular belief, is a recent addition to Asian diets. The milk has a natural unpleasant odour and taste because of the presence of compounds produced by the enzyme lipooxygenase. For this reason, soy milk is often loaded with sweeteners and artificial flavours, or more often, it is made from isolated soy proteins combined with other ingredients. If you're looking for high-quality soy milk, make sure you read the labels before making a purchase.

A WHOLE GRAIN OF TRUTH

So You Say You Want a Revolution?

Cereals and pseudo-cereals provide the majority of calories and carbohydrates to the world's human population. The top eight cereal grains—wheat, maize, rice, barley, sorghum, oats, rye and millet—provide 56% of the food energy and half of the protein consumed on earth. Only three cereals—wheat, maize and rice—comprise at least 87% of the world's grain production. Humans have become so dependent on cereal grains that one researcher pointed out, "cereal grains literally stand between mankind and starvation." This is no exaggeration. The agricultural system that is in place today is a result of the Green Revolution, a series of highly orchestrated, global strategies developed in the face of looming starvation. This huge international effort began in the 1960s and achieved adequacy in world food calorie and protein production in just two decades, an impressive effort for which one of the leaders received the Nobel Peace Prize. In the last 50 years, the average yield per unit of land of cereals has increased by more than 50%.

Compared with other crops, cereals and pseudo-cereals can be stored for many years without a serious loss of quality, which can supply the masses with a steady supply of calories between seasonal harvests. This characteristic allowed our Paleolithic ancestors to adopt agriculture and eschew their nomadic ways in favour of settlement and food security. Grains provided more food with less effort than any other crop, allowing more time for people to develop other pursuits. This newfound time led to social stratification that was ultimately responsible for the vast technological and industrial culture in which we live today. The enormous advances in knowledge and understanding of medicine, science and the universe would never have been possible had it not been for the widespread adoption of cereal agriculture by humanity.

Agriculture, however, is a double-edged sword. During the Green Revolution's push toward food security, little thought was given to nutritional value and human health. Grains are an excellent source of B vitamins and energy, but they are deficient in some amino acids and micronutrients such as iron. As the production of cereal grains in developing countries increased, they displaced traditional crops that were more nutrient-rich, causing widespread micronutrient deficiencies, often called "hidden hunger." Nevertheless, the prospect of mass starvation, inevitable without the Green Revolution, is far worse than the problems that now need to be addressed.

Cereals and Pseudo-cereals

Cereals, derived from the name of the Roman goddess of harvest and agriculture Ceres, belong to the grass family. Pseudo-cereals belong to other botanical families and, like cereals, are grown for their edible starchy seeds. An example is quinoa from the Amaranth family. Unlike cereals, pseudo-cereals contain all essential amino acids for humans, making them a complete protein. This quality is usually rare in plants. Cereals are deficient in the essential amino acid lysine, which is why vegetarian cultures combine it with pseudo-cereals or legumes.

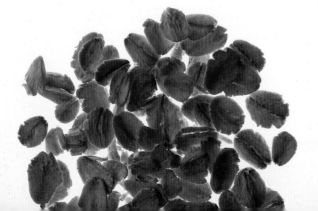

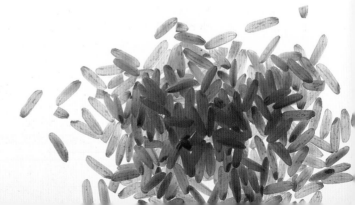

Our Moral Fibre

Grains are seeds that contain three parts: the bran, the endosperm and the germ. Whole grains, such as rolled oats and brown rice, contain all three parts of the kernel. Refined grains, such as white rice, white flour and cream of wheat, have the bran and endosperm removed, resulting in the loss of fibre, vitamins and minerals. In Canada, manufacturers are required to enrich white flour with some of the lost vitamins, but it still lacks fibre and some other nutrients. Research has shown that whole grain and pseudo-grain consumption helps lower the risk of cardiovascular disease, stroke, type 2 diabetes, metabolic syndrome and gastrointestinal cancers. In the Physician's Health Study, researchers followed more than 21,000 participants over a 20-year period and found that men who consumed a morning bowl of whole grain (but not refined) cereal had a 29% lower risk of heart failure. Significant cardiovascular benefits were also observed in postmenopausal women who consumed at least six servings of whole grains per week over a period of three years. In the UK Women's Cohort Study, which included close to 36,000 participants, pre-menopausal women who ate at least 13 grams of whole grain fibre per day had a 41% reduced risk of breast cancer compared to those who only ate 4 g or less per day.

The Other Guys

Beyond fibre, researchers have found that whole grains and pseudo-cereals contain some powerful phenolic compounds that have antioxidant properties and can protect against degenerative diseases. Most of the scientific literature on plant phenolics has focused on those in fruits, vegetables, wines and teas. However, many of these same phenolics are also reported in cereals but have been overlooked because most of the focus had been on the fibre content. The phytochemical content of cereals may explain why some studies have shown that populations eating diets high in fibre-rich whole grains consistently have lower risk of colon cancer, yet short-term clinical trials that have focused on fibre alone often yielded inconsistent results. Some phenolic compounds are unique among gains species. Oats for example, contain avenanthamides, antioxidant compounds that reduce inflammation and reduce the risk of atherosclerosis. In the bran of barley, wheat and rye, alkylresorcinols have been shown to possess potent anti-bacterial and anti-fungal activity. Lignans found in barley, oats and rye are converted to phytoestrogens by our microbial flora and are believed to reduce the risk of hormone-dependent cancers, colon cancer and heart disease.

Grainy Outlook

Cereal grains have always been associated with life and culture. They are featured on the flags of several major countries, carved into the stonework of churches and cemeteries, and are an important component of various rituals and ceremonies. Grain production was so important to the Romans that the primary concern of Ceres was the protection of grain. Enjoy whole cereals and pseudo-cereals as part of your healthy way of eating. These superfoods can significantly lower your risk of several chronic diseases and can easily be stored in your cupboard to eat at your convenience.

Barley

Although it is a staple in many Middle Eastern diets, barley hasn't enjoyed the same popularity in North America, where it is primarily used as livestock feed and in the production of beer. The most common forms of barley available in the supermarket are pearl barley, which has been polished to remove the outer hull, bran and some of the endosperm layer, and pot barley, which has the outer hull removed but the other layers intact. Choose pot barley to get more nutritional bang for your buck. Barley is an excellent source of fibre, which helps lower cholesterol, prevent heart disease and provides a measure of protection against colon cancer and hemorrhoids. It is also a good source of selenium, iron, vitamin B6 and folate.

Corn, Barley and Bean Soup

Serves 6 to 8

½ cup (125 mL) barley

¼ tsp (1 mL) canola oil

1 large onion, chopped

½ cup (125 mL) chopped celery

½ cup (125 mL) chopped carrots

1 clove garlic, minced

½ tsp (2 mL) dried basil

½ tsp (2 mL) dried oregano

1 bay leaf

8 cups (2 L) vegetable stock

2 cups (500 mL) corn kernels

1½ cups (375 mL) cooked beans, such as cannellini

1 cup (250 mL) julienned leafy greens

½ tsp (2 mL) each salt and pepper

Heat a medium saucepan over medium. Add barley to pan and cook, stirring constantly, until barley is golden and smells nutty, about 3 minutes. Transfer barley to a plate and return pan to heat. Add oil to pan and heat. Add onion, celery, carrot and garlic. Cook until onion has softened, about 2 minutes. Add barley, basil, oregano, bay leaf and stock. Bring to a boil. Reduce heat to medium-low. Simmer until barley is *al dente*, about 20 minutes. Remove bay leaf. Stir in corn, beans, greens, salt and pepper. Continue cooking until hot.

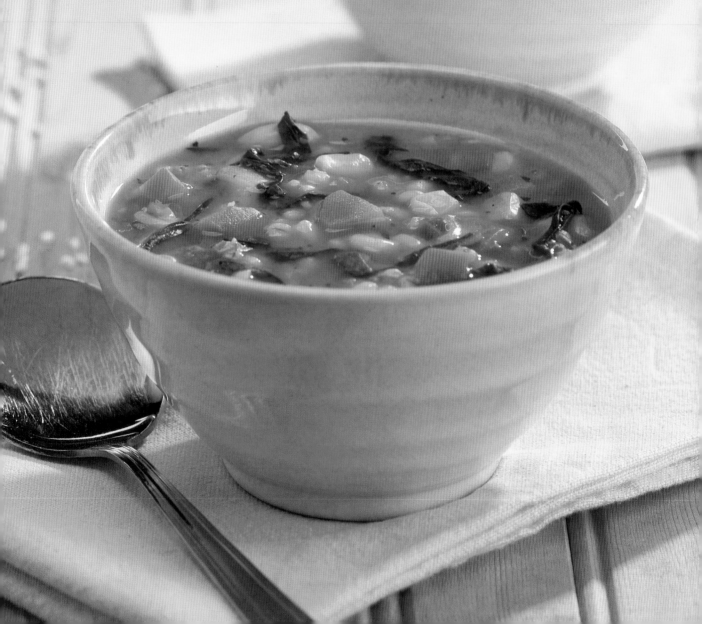

In Rome's first cookbook, *De Re Coquinaria, the author, Apicius, made a complex broth by soaking barley a full day before cooking it with oil, dill, onions, salt and herbs and spices such as coriander, lovage, cumin and pepper. Pliny the Elder wrote about oily barley bread seasoned with coriander. No doubt he was looking over Apicius' shoulder.*

Toasted Barley Risotto

Serves 4

4 cups (1 L) vegetable stock, *divided*

1 cup (250 mL) pearl barley

1 tsp (5 mL) canola oil

½ cup (125 mL) finely chopped onion

3 cloves garlic, minced

1 bay leaf

2 tsp (10 mL) chopped fresh oregano

2 tsp (10 mL) finely grated lemon zest

1 tsp (5 mL) chopped fresh thyme

⅛ tsp (0.5 mL) sea salt

pinch of pepper

up to 1 cup (250 mL) steamed or sautéed vegetables of your choice, optional

Heat stock in a medium saucepan over medium-high until hot, then reduce heat to medium-low to keep warm.

Heat a medium saucepan over medium. Add barley to pan and cook, stirring constantly, until barley is golden and smells nutty, about 3 minutes. Transfer barley to a bowl and return pan to heat. Add oil to pan and heat. Add onion and garlic. Cook until onion has softened, about 2 minutes. Add barley and cook, stirring, for 1 minute. Add bay leaf. Stir in ½ cup (125 mL) warm stock and cook, stirring until absorbed. Continue adding warm stock ½ cup (125 mL) at a time until barley is tender, about 20 to 30 minutes.

Stir in oregano, lemon zest, thyme, salt, pepper and vegetables, if using. Remove bay leaf before serving.

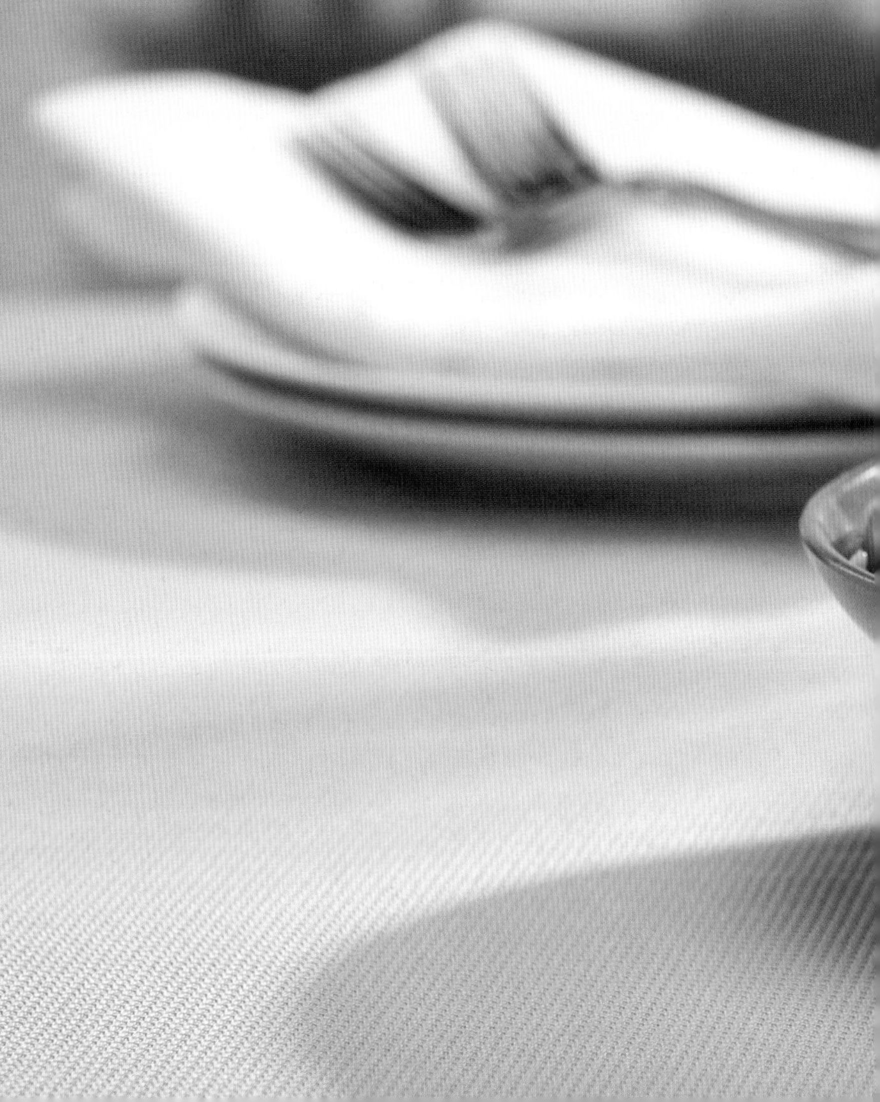

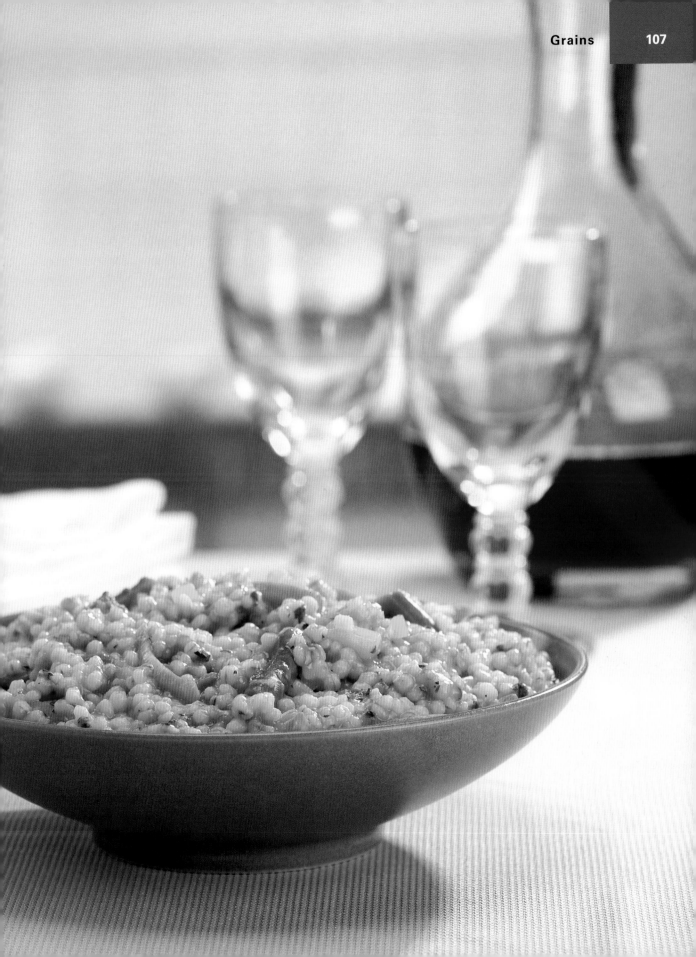

Oats

What makes oats a superstar among cereals is their fibre content. Oats contain a nice mix of both soluble and insoluble fibre, but it is the type of soluble fibre, called beta-glucan, that is responsible for most of oats' health benefits. Beta-glucan can help lower LDL cholesterol, reduce the rick of cardiovascular disease and stroke, and boost the immune system. Oats are also a good source of protein and have a low glycemic load, meaning that they do not have a large affect on blood sugar, making them a good choice of grain for people who are diabetic. Most supermarkets carry both steel-cut oats, which are simply oats that have been cut into a few pieces, and rolled oats, which are somewhat more processed and have been flattened and steamed or lightly toasted; both are healthy choices. Avoid instant rolled oats, which are less nutritious and can be chock-full of added sugar.

Good for You Granola

Makes about 10 cups (2.5 L)

6 cups (1.5 L) large flake rolled oats

3 cups (750 mL) oat bran

¼ cup (60 mL) hulled raw pumpkin seeds

¼ cup (60 mL) hulled raw sunflower seeds

1 cup (250 mL) agave nectar or raw honey

1 vanilla bean, split

Preheat oven to 400° F (200° C). Divide rolled oats and oat bran among 2 baking sheets and spread evenly. Toast until golden, about 5 to 8 minutes.

Spread pumpkin seeds and sunflower seeds evenly on a third baking sheet. Toast, stirring once or twice, until lightly browned, about 5 minutes.

Place agave nectar or honey in a small saucepan. Scrape seeds from vanilla bean into pan and reserve pod for another use. Cook over low heat to infuse agave nectar with vanilla flavour, about 5 to 7 minutes.

(continued on next page)

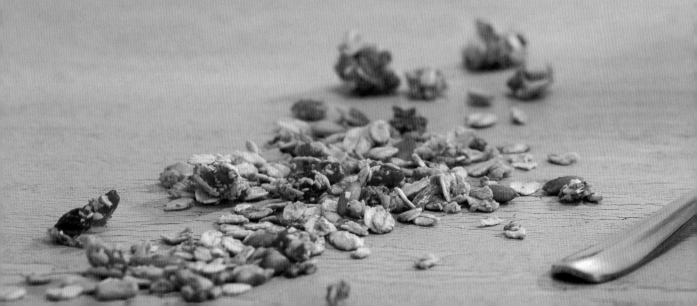

Bring apple juice to a simmer in a medium saucepan. Turn off heat, add dried fruit, cover and let sit about 10 minutes to soften fruit. Drain fruit, reserving any remaining liquid for another use (e.g., add to a smoothie). Combine toasted oats, oat bran and seeds with fruit mixture in a large bowl. Add warm agave nectar and stir to coat as evenly as possible. Divide mixture among 2 baking sheets. Bake, stirring frequently, until golden, about 10 to 15 minutes. Cool completely before transferring to an airtight container to store at room temperature for up to 1 month.

3 cups (750 mL) unsweetened apple juice

½ cup (125 mL) dried goji berries

½ cup (125 mL) raisins

½ cup (125 mL) chopped dates

Middle age is when you choose your cereal for the fibre, not the toy.

—Unknown

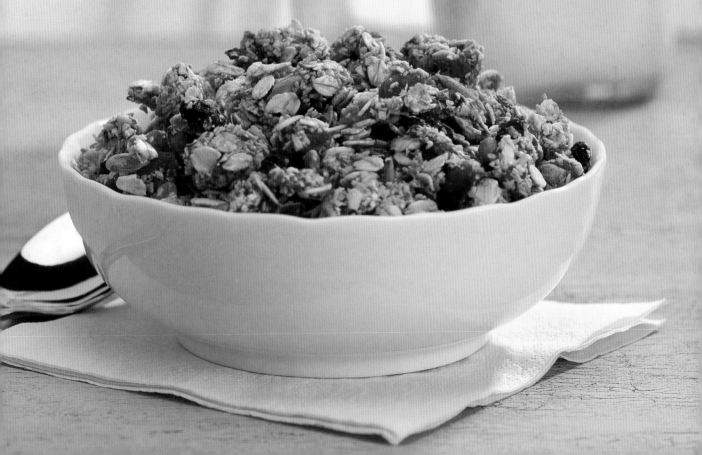

Multi-grain Baked Apples

Serves 4

½ cup (125 mL) large flake rolled oats

2 Tbsp (30 mL) butter

⅓ cup (75 mL) cooked wild rice

⅛ tsp (0.5 mL) stevia concentrate powder

1 tsp (5 mL) grated lemon zest

½ tsp (2 mL) gound cinnamon

½ tsp (2 mL) ground nutmeg

4 large unpeeled apples, such as Golden Delicious

1 cup (250 mL) apple juice

Heat small sauté pan on medium. Add oats and cook for about 5 minutes, stirring occasionally, until lightly browned. Add butter. Heat, stirring, until melted. Add wild rice, stevia, lemon zest, cinnamon and nutmeg. Heat, stirring, for 1 minute, then set aside. Carefully remove cores from apples using a melon baller, to about ½ in (12 mm) from bottom. Fill apples with oat mixture. Pour apple juice into a 2 quart (2 L) deep casserole. Place apples in juice and bake, covered, in 375° F (190° C) oven for 30 to 35 minutes until apples are tender when pierced with a fork.

Oats. A grain, which in England is generally given to horses, but in Scotland supports the people.

—Samuel Johnson

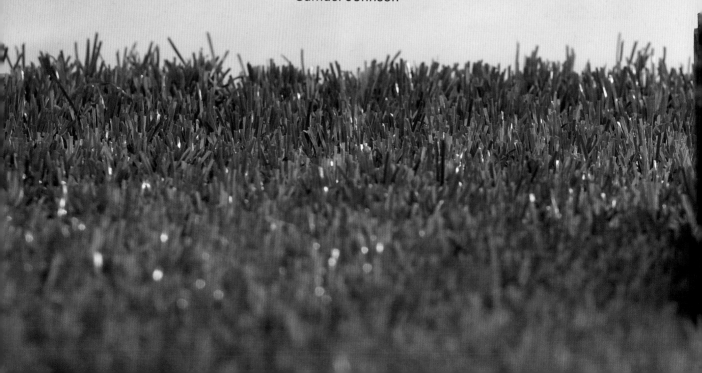

Stevia contains steviol glycosides, which are 300 times sweeter than sugar. Because stevia has a negligible effect on blood sugar and has zero calories, it is attractive to both food manufacturers and consumers. Stevia's sweetness has a slower onset and longer duration than sugar, but some extracts leave a slightly bitter aftertaste that some find disagreeable. The plant has been used for more than 1500 years by the Guaraní people of Paraguay and Brazil to sweeten their *yerba mate (a tea-like beverage)* and as a medicine to treat heartburn and other ailments.

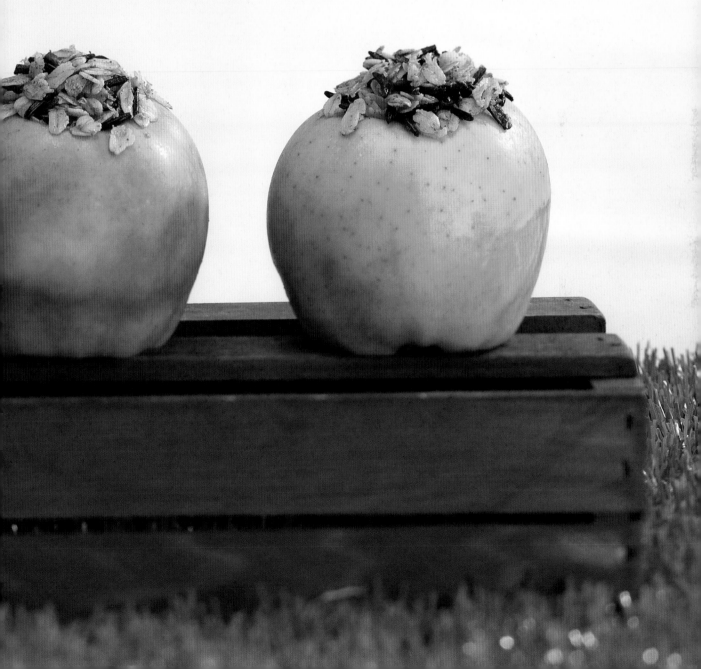

Quinoa

Quinoa is a staple that has been cultivated in the Andean mountain regions of Peru, Chile and Bolivia for over 5000 years and was once called "mother of all grains." Early Spanish colonists forbade quinoa cultivation because of its association with non-Christian Indians. In the 1980s, the nutritional value of quinoa was recognized, and it has since become more available to North Americans. Quinoa is higher in protein than any other grain and is also a complete protein, meaning that it contains all essential amino acids. It is an excellent source of iron and fibre and a good source of calcium, folate and magnesium. The United Nations has even classified quinoa as a supercrop because it is such a complete foodstuff. And unlike some cereals, quinoa does not contain gluten, a protein found in wheat, barley and rye that has an adverse effect in those that are sensitive and prone to celiac disease.

Quinoa-crusted Salmon with Citrus Sauce

Serves 4

1½ cups (375 mL) freshly squeezed orange juice

¼ cup (60 mL) minced ginger

¼ cup (60 mL) tamari

2 Tbsp (30 mL) lemon juice

4 tsp (20 mL) lime juice

2 tsp (10 mL) sesame oil

Preheat oven to 400° F (200° C). Combine orange juice, ginger, tamari, lemon juice and lime juice in a medium saucepan. Bring to a boil on medium-high, then reduce heat to medium and simmer, uncovered, until reduced by half, about 15 minutes. Pour through a fine-mesh sieve, then discard solids and stir in sesame oil.

(continued on next page)

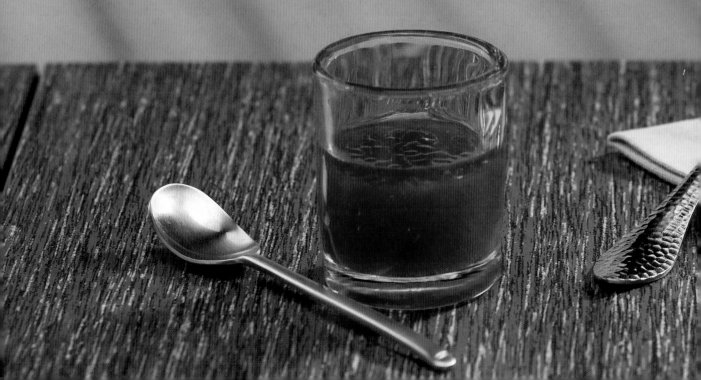

Meanwhile, pour quinoa onto a plate. Pat salmon dry and sprinkle lightly with salt and pepper. Press salmon firmly into quinoa to coat all sides.

Heat canola oil in a large oven-safe sauté pan over medium. Add salmon and fry until quinoa is golden, about 2 to 3 minutes on each side. Transfer to oven and bake until cooked through, about 6 minutes. Transfer to serving plates and pour sauce around fillets.

½ cup (125 mL) quinoa

4 x 4 to 6 oz (115 to 170 g) skinless salmon fillets

sea salt and pepper

1 Tbsp (15 mL) canola oil

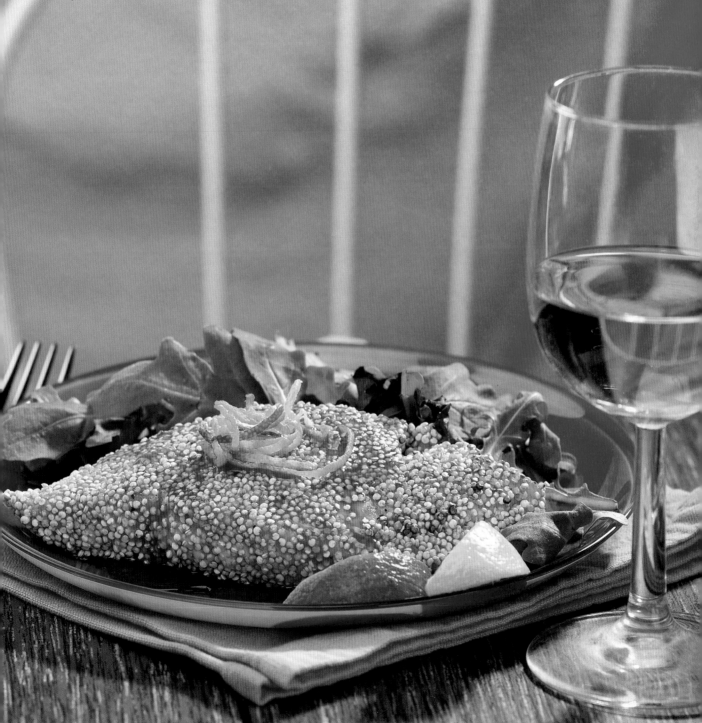

Quinoa Salad

Serves 6 as a main course

juice from 1 lemon

⅓ cup (75 mL) apple cider vinegar

½ cup (125 mL) orange juice

⅓ cup (75 mL) canola or sunflower oil

⅓ cup (75 mL) honey

4 cups (1 L) cooked quinoa (see Tip)

2 apples such as Honeycrisp or Gala, cored and chopped

1 bell pepper, diced small

1 cup (250 mL) fresh corn kernels

½ cup (125 mL) dried cranberries

½ cup (125 mL) currants

1 small red onion, finely chopped

1 cup (250 mL) chopped pecans, toasted

1 cup (250 mL) fresh parsley and mint, chopped

sea salt and freshly ground pepper to taste

Place lemon juice, apple cider vinegar, orange juice, oil and honey in a small bowl and stir to combine. In a large bowl, combine quinoa, apple, bell pepper, corn, cranberries, currants, onion, pecans and parsley, then stir in dressing. Add salt and pepper to taste and refrigerate until ready to serve.

Tip

To cook quinoa, bring 4 cups (1 L) water to a boil in a wide-bottomed pot with a lid. Add a pinch of salt and stir in 2 cups (500 mL) quinoa. Reduce heat to a simmer, cover and cook until all the water has absorbed, about 25 minutes. You can cook any amount of quinoa you like as long as you keep the 2:1 ratio of liquid to grain. It is also worth experimenting with other liquids such as stock or coconut milk.

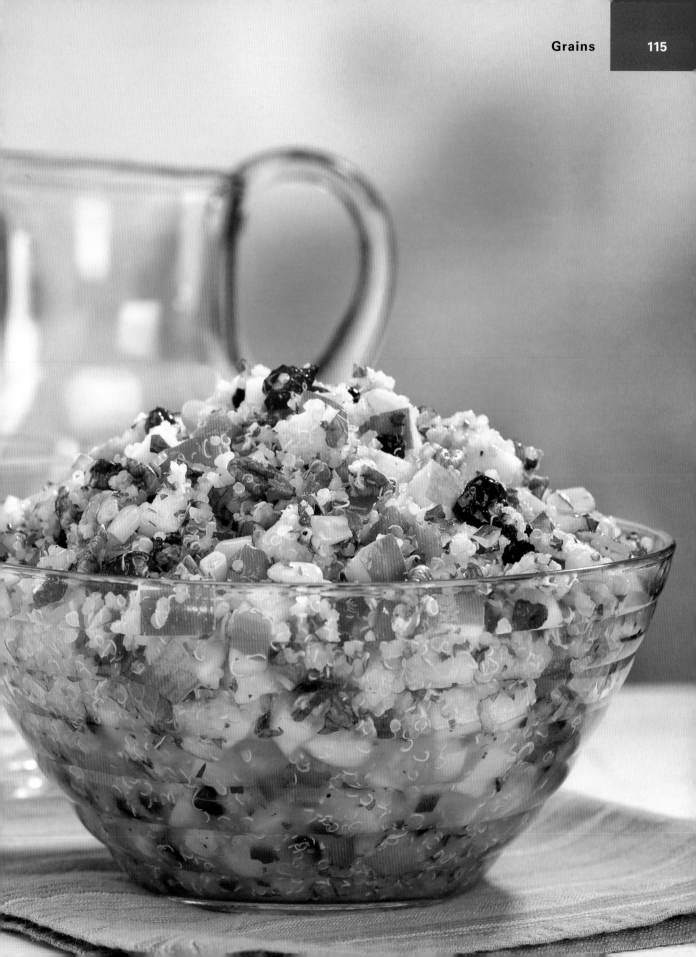

Brown Rice

Although rice is a staple of cultures around the world, the majority of what is eaten is white rice. White rice is simply brown rice that has been stripped of the outer hull and bran layer. This process shortens the rice's cooking time and extends the shelf life (brown rice goes rancid much quicker than white) but it also robs the rice of most of its nutrients. Brown rice, however, still has the bran layer intact and therefore still contains much of its nutrition. Brown rice is an excellent source of vitamin B6 and is high in niacin, magnesium, manganese and phosphorus. It is also a good source of insoluble fibre, which protects against colon cancer, and selenium, a mineral that inhibits the growth of cancer cells and induces their apoptosis.

Brown Rice Quinoa Pilaf

Makes 8 cups (2 L)

1 Tbsp (15 mL) canola oil

1 cup (250 mL) finely chopped onion

1 cup (250 mL) grated carrot

1 cup (250 mL) long grain brown rice

3½ cups (875 mL) vegetable stock

1 cup (250 mL) quinoa, rinsed and drained

½cup (125 mL) dried cranberries

Heat oil in a large saucepan over medium. Add onion and carrot. Cook, uncovered, for 5 to 10 minutes, stirring often, until onion has softened. Add rice and stir until coated. Stir in stock, and bring to a boil. Reduce heat to medium-low and simmer, covered, for 20 minutes, without stirring. Stir in quinoa and cranberries, and bring to a boil. Reduce heat to medium-low and simmer, covered, for 20 to 25 minutes more, again without stirring, until rice and quinoa are tender and stock has absorbed.

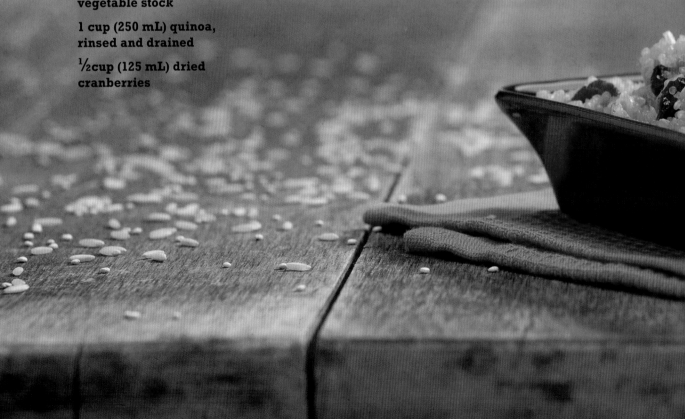

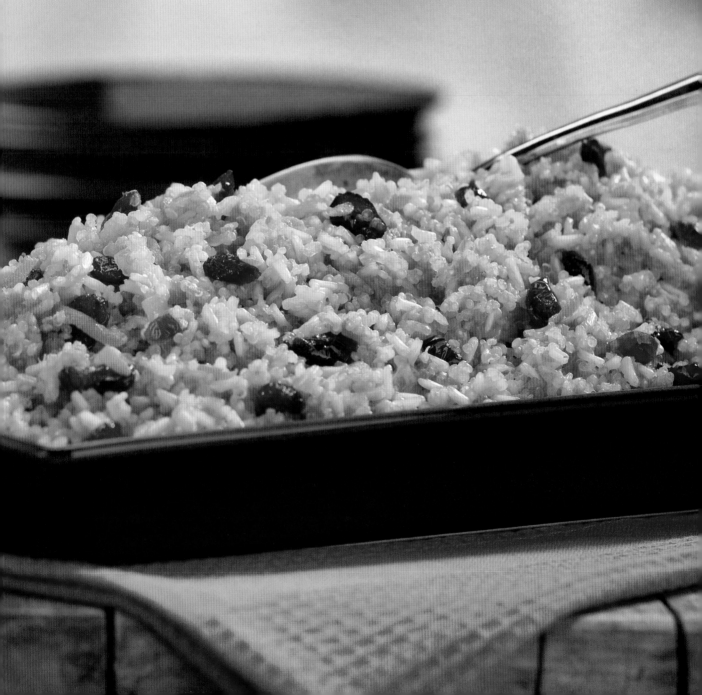

I like rice. Rice is great if you're hungry and want 2000 of something.

—Mitch Hedberg

Edamame Fried Rice

Serves 6

¼ tsp (1 mL) canola oil

1 egg, lightly beaten

1 Tbsp (15 mL) chopped onion

½ tsp (2 mL) minced ginger

½ tsp (2 mL) minced garlic

1 Tbsp (15 mL) chopped celery

1 Tbsp (15 mL) chopped red or orange bell pepper

1 Tbsp (15 mL) chopped broccoli

2 Tbsp (30 mL) chopped snow peas

½ cup (125 mL) edamame

2 cups (500 mL) cooked brown rice

2 Tbsp (30 mL) shredded carrot

1 Tbsp (15 mL) chopped green onion

1 Tbsp (15 mL) soy sauce

Heat oil in a medium sauté pan over medium. Add egg and cook, stirring gently, until scrambled. Transfer to a small bowl and set aside. In same pan, add onion, ginger, garlic, celery, bell pepper, broccoli, snow peas and edamame and cook, stirring, for about 2 minutes, until onion has softened. Stir in rice and carrot and cook for about 3 minutes, until rice is heated through. Remove from heat and add egg, green onion, and soy sauce.

With coarse rice to eat, with water to drink, and my bent arm for a pillow—I have still joy in the midst of all these things.

—Confucius

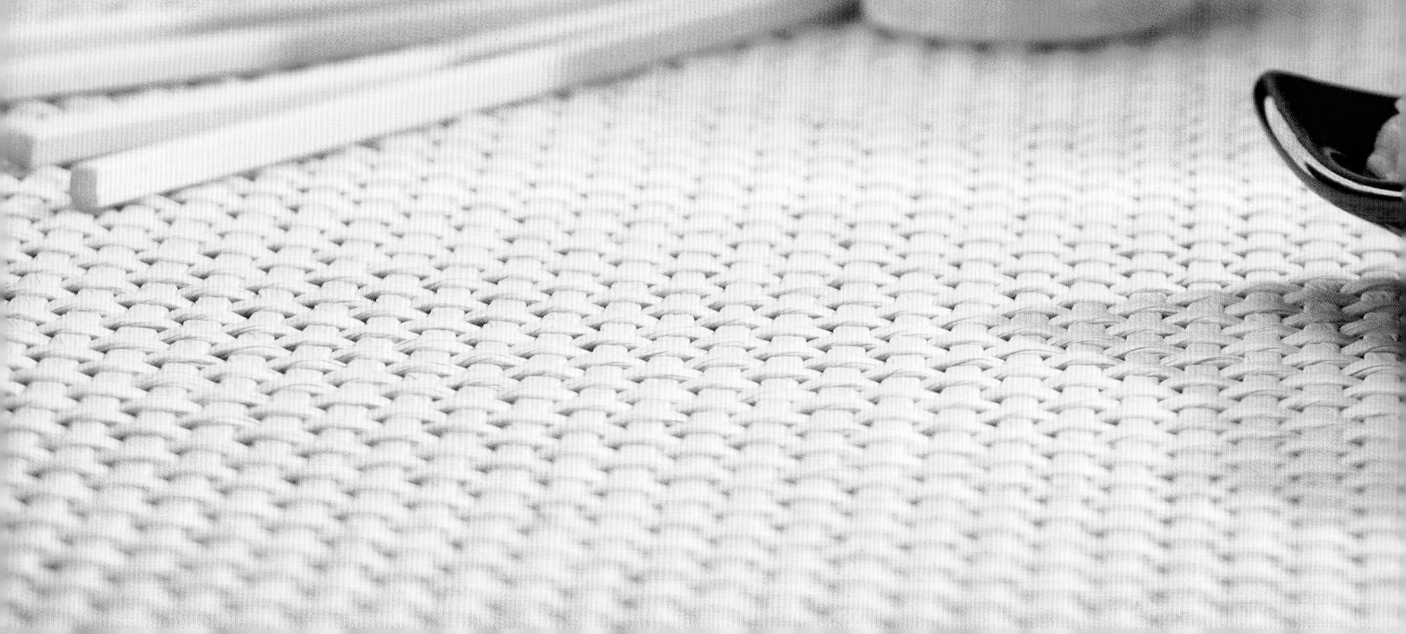

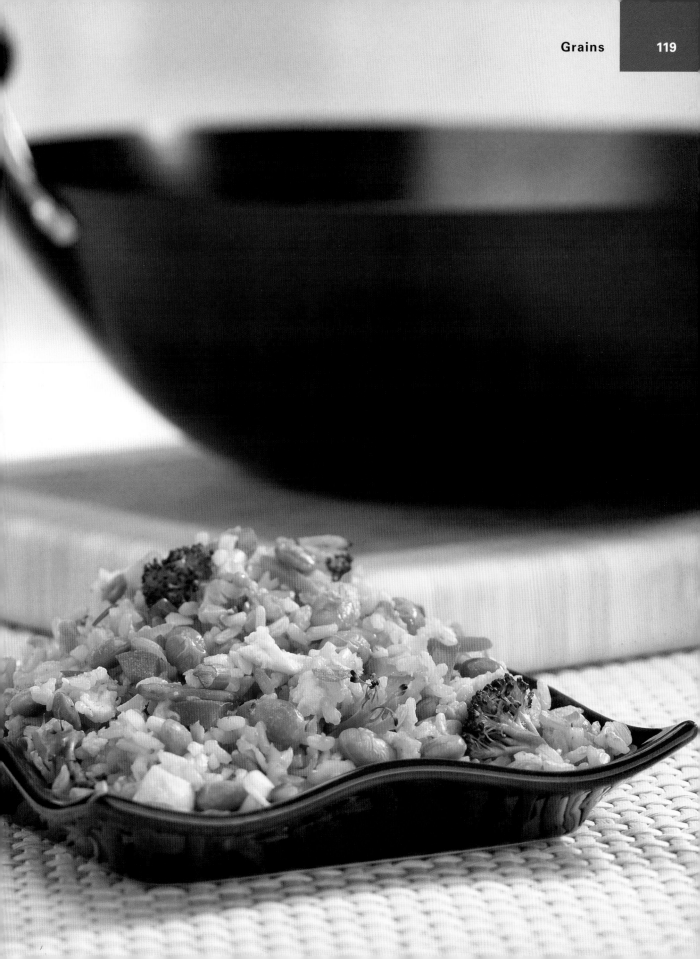

THE NUTS AND BOLTS OF SEEDS AND NUTS

Nut Case

"You're nuts," "what a nut-job," "you belong in a nuthouse," "check out that nutter," "you're a real nutcase"—how did nuts become so synonymous with craziness? In the mid-1800s, the word "nut" was slang for head, so if someone said you were off your nut, it meant you were crazy. Another possibility is that in the late 1800s, the British used nuts as a slang for something that was enjoyable, as in "I'm nuts about you." But this could also be reworded as "I'm crazy about you," so it didn't take much to interchange the meaning of the two. In the *New Oxford American Dictionary*, the noun "nut" is explained as: "[informal] a person's head" or "[informal] a crazy or eccentric person." The term is well established in our vernacular and continues to appear in movies, songs, advertisements and everyday conversations. After you learn of all the incredible health benefits that nuts have to offer, you'll go nuts over them.

Health Nut

Botanically speaking, a true nut is a hard-shelled fruit that has one seed, like a hazelnut or chestnut. Most of the things we think of as being nuts are actually not. Almonds, pecans, pistachios and walnuts are all seeds of drupe fruits, like peaches and plums, which have the leathery flesh removed at harvest; the peanut is a legume like the bean; macadamia nuts are kernels; pine nuts are the seeds of conifers; Brazil nuts are the seeds from a capsule; and cashews are seeds of a drupe that grow at the end of a fleshy fruit. Flaxseeds are well, seeds, that have a nutty flavour and have very similar nutritional qualities to nuts. Regardless of whether they're true nuts, fake nuts or just plain nuts, they are nutritional powerhouses that can significantly improve your heart health. A handful or two of nuts every day can lower your low-density lipoprotein (LDL) levels and reduce your risk of having a heart attack.

All large prospective cohort studies that have examined the relation between nut consumption and the risk or coronary heart disease (the Iowa Women Health Study, the Nurses' Health Study, the Physician's Health Study and the CARE Study) have found a significant inverse association. The Nurses' Health Study found that substituting 1 oz (28 g) of nuts for carbohydrates in an average diet would reduce coronary heart disease risk by about 30%, and substitution for saturated fat would decrease it further to 45%. The evidence for the beneficial effects of nuts is so strong that it seems justifiable to move them to a more prominent place in our diets.

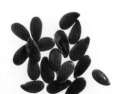
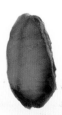
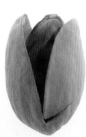

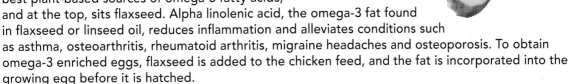

Fat Chance

Nuts have a high fat content but should not be spurned by those who are fat phobic. The beneficial effects of nuts underscore the importance of distinguishing different types of fat. The mono- and polyunsaturated fats are considered "good" fats that help reduce LDL cholesterol levels. Nuts (especially walnuts) are also rich in omega-3 fatty acids, which have a stellar reputation for being healthy. Nuts are one of the best plant-based sources of omega-3 fatty acids, and at the top, sits flaxseed. Alpha linolenic acid, the omega-3 fat found in flaxseed or linseed oil, reduces inflammation and alleviates conditions such as asthma, osteoarthritis, rheumatoid arthritis, migraine headaches and osteoporosis. To obtain omega-3 enriched eggs, flaxseed is added to the chicken feed, and the fat is incorporated into the growing egg before it is hatched.

Among the fats found in nuts and flax is vitamin E, an essential fat-soluble antioxidant that halts the development of arterial plaques and prevents coronary artery disease. Research shows that a mere 2 oz (55 g) a day of pistachios can significantly boost blood levels of gamma-tocopherol, a natural form of vitamin E, that may offer protection against lung, prostate, and possibly other forms of cancer.

Nut fat also contains phytosterols that are able to reduce blood levels of total and LDL cholesterol by competing with dietary and biliary cholesterol for absorption in the intestine. In a study involving 40 patients with high cholesterol, consuming 0.7 oz (20 g) of ground flaxseed for two months reduced total cholesterol, LDL cholesterol, triglycerides and the ratio of total to HDL cholesterol to the same extent as those who were given statin drugs.

A little goes a long way

It's easy to include nuts in your diet. Enjoy them as snacks, sprinkled in salads, blended in smoothies, ground into salad dressings, or included in baked goods. If you want to receive the maximum health benefits from nuts, buy them raw and keep them in the refrigerator for freshness. To roast them, do so at low temperatures to minimize the loss of antioxidants. Place them on a baking sheet and dry-roast them at 65 to 75° C for 15 to 20 minutes, then transfer to a dish to cool. As few as 1 to 3 oz (28 to 85 g) of nuts a day will have potent benefits for your health. That translates to two generous handfuls of nuts, which just happens to correspond to the number of hands we were born with. Coincidence?

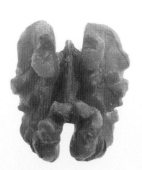
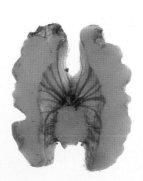
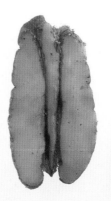
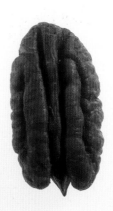

Flaxseed

Flaxseed's species name is *usitatissimum,* meaning "most useful," which would accurately describe the nutritional and medicinal value of this tiny nutty seed. An ancient Mesopotamian plant known since the Stone Age, its popularity waned after the fall of the Roman Empire, though Charlemagne was so impressed with the versatility of its uses, including its fibres that can be woven into linen, that he passed laws requiring not only its cultivation but also its consumption. Flaxseed has been receiving some interest recently because of its special ability to protect women's health. The plant is particularly rich in lignin, compounds that are converted by gut microflora to two hormone-like compounds called enterolactone and enterdiol. Their weak estrogenic activity offers protection against breast cancer in post-menopausal women without interfering with estrogen's role in normal bone maintenance. Flax may also be beneficial for reducing hot flashes. Postmenopausal women who suffered at least 14 hot flashes per week had 50% less episodes after eating 1.5 oz (40 g) of crushed flaxseed every day for six weeks. Note that the lignans are found in the flaxseed, not in the oil, and remember to grind the seeds just prior to consuming them or they will be difficult to digest.

Seed and Fruit Granola Bars

Makes 12 bars

2 cups (500 mL) large flake rolled oats

½ cup (125 mL) raw pumpkin seeds

½ cup (125 mL) raw sunflower seeds

⅓ cup (75 mL) chopped dried cherries

⅓ cup (75 mL) dried blueberries

⅓ cup (75 mL) golden raisins

⅓ cup (75 mL) wheat germ

1 Tbsp (15 mL) flaxseed

1 Tbsp (15 mL) sesame seeds

Spread rolled oats on an ungreased rimmed baking sheet. Bake in 350° F (175° C) oven for about 18 minutes, stirring occasionally, until golden. Transfer to a large bowl.

Stir in pumpkin seeds, sunflower seeds, cherries, blueberries, raisins, wheat germ, flaxseed and sesame seeds.

(continued on next page)

Combine butter, sugar (or stevia), honey and maple syrup in a small saucepan. Heat and stir on medium for about 5 minutes until starting to boil. Drizzle over rolled oat mixture and stir until coated. Press into a greased 9 x 13 in (23 x 33 cm) pan. Bake for about 15 minutes until golden. Let stand for 15 minutes to cool slightly. Run knife around inside edge of pan to loosen. Cut into 12 bars while still warm. Let stand in pan on wire rack until cool.

$1/3$ cup (75 mL) butter

$1/4$ cup (60 mL) muscovado sugar, packed (or 2 tsp [10 mL]) stevia powder)

$1/4$ cup (60 mL) liquid honey

$1/4$ cup (60 mL) maple syrup

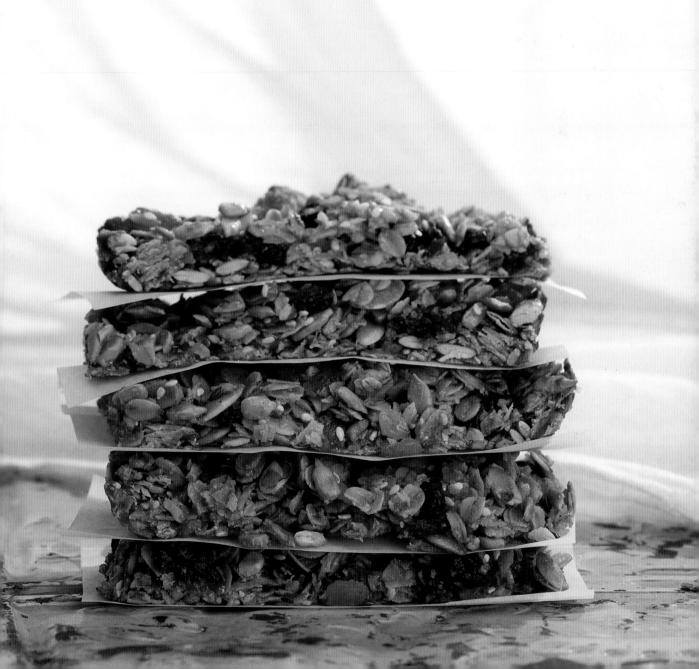

Fruited Muesli

Makes 6 cups (1.5 L)

½ cup (125 mL) apple juice

½ cup (125 mL) water

1 cup (250 mL) large flake rolled oats

2 cups (500 mL) chopped, unpeeled apple, such as McIntosh

2 cups (500 mL) plain yogurt

½ cup (125 mL) chopped dried apricot

½ cup (125 mL) raisins

¼ cup (60 mL) ground flaxseed (see Tip)

¼ cup (60 mL) sliced almonds, toasted

¼ cup (60 mL) unsalted, roasted sunflower seeds

3 Tbsp (45 mL) maple syrup

1 tsp (5 mL) grated orange zest

1 tsp (5 mL) cinnamon

Combine apple juice and water in a medium saucepan. Bring to a boil, then remove from heat. Stir in oats, and transfer to a medium bowl. Chill for 25 to 30 minutes until liquid has absorbed. Stir in apple, yogurt, apricot, raisins, flaxseed, almonds, sunflower seeds, maple syrup, zest and cinnamon.

Tip

Grind 2½ Tbsp (37 mL) whole flaxseed in blender or coffee grinder to yield ¼ cup (60 mL) ground flaxseed.

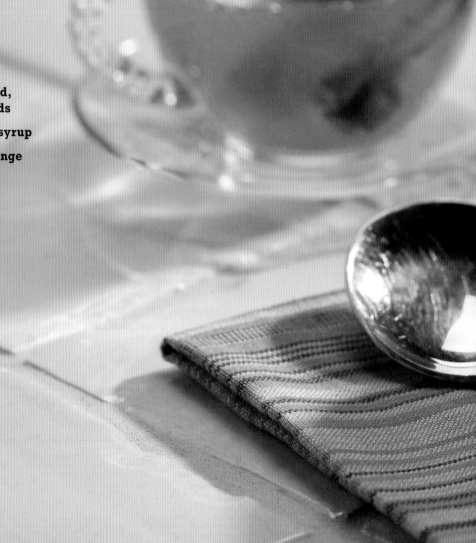

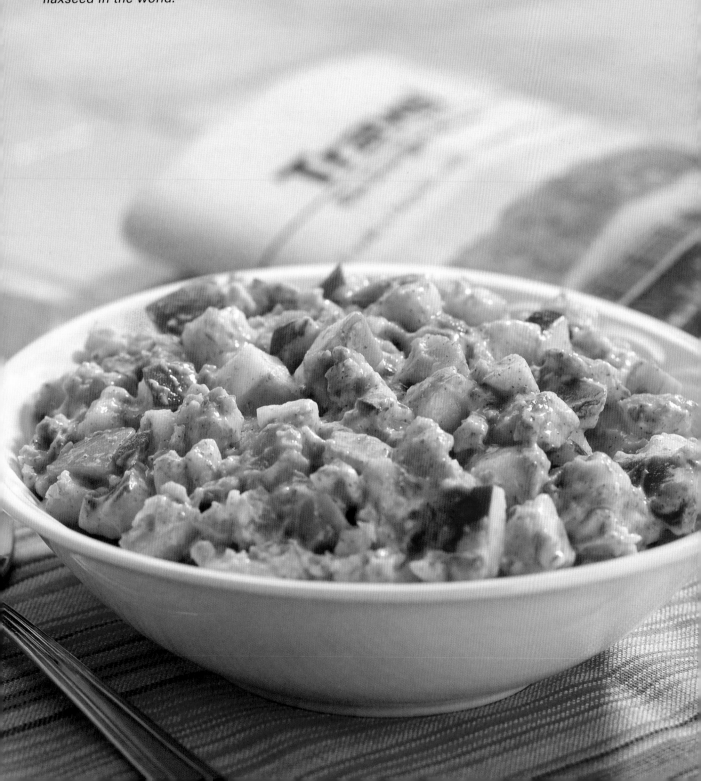

Flaxseeds weren't introduced to Canada until the 1600s, but the country is now the largest producer of flaxseed in the world.

Tree Nuts

Tree nuts contain an arsenal of powerful antioxidants that can scavenge harmful free radicals and reduce oxidative damage to cellular membranes. In a small study of only 13 participants, a walnut or almond smoothie was given every day after an overnight fast and after a week, researchers found a noticeable increase in blood levels of antioxidant polyphenols, an increase in total antioxidant capacity and a decrease in blood oxidation levels compared to nut-free smoothies. In another small study with 16 participants, meals including whole and blended pecans caused a decrease in LDL oxidation, a decrease in levels of triglycerides and an increase in antioxidant levels. In almonds, 20 different antioxidant flavonoids, some of which were the same as those found in green tea and grapefruit, were found in the almond skin. Researchers found that the skins prevented LDL oxidation by 18%, but when tested together with the vitamin E in the meat of the almond, resistance to oxidation increased by 52%. So next time you eat almonds, make sure to eat them whole, including the skin. Of all the antioxidant-rich nuts, the undeniable nut king is the walnut, probably because it is usually consumed raw and unroasted. Many nuts are commercially roasted in added fats and at high temperatures that damage and reduce antioxidant levels. To get the full effectiveness of nut antioxidants, make sure to eat more walnuts as part of a healthy diet.

Raw Chocolate Almond Fudge

Makes 16 squares

1 cup (250 mL) coconut oil

½ cup (125 mL) almond butter

1 cup (250 mL) raw cacao powder

1 cup (250 mL) agave nectar

1 Tbsp (15 mL) vanilla

¼ tsp (1 mL) sea salt

¼ tsp (1 mL) cinnamon

½ cup (125 mL) almonds

Cream together coconut oil and almond butter in a large bowl until smooth. Add cacao and mix until fully incorporated. Add agave nectar, vanilla, salt and cinnamon. Mix until smooth, stopping and scraping down sides of bowl, mashing any lumps against sides if necessary. Stir in almonds and mix until evenly distributed. Pour into a 7 x 11 in (18 cm x 28 cm) glass dish. Freeze until firm, about 1 to 2 hours. Cut into squares. Store, covered, in refrigerator for up to 1 week or in freezer up to 1 month.

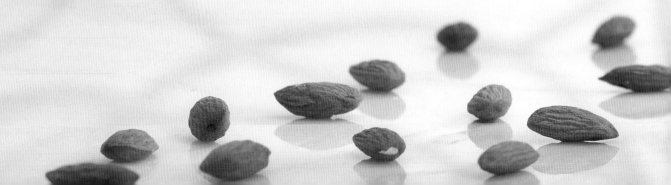

You must crack the nut before you can eat the kernel.

—Irish proverb

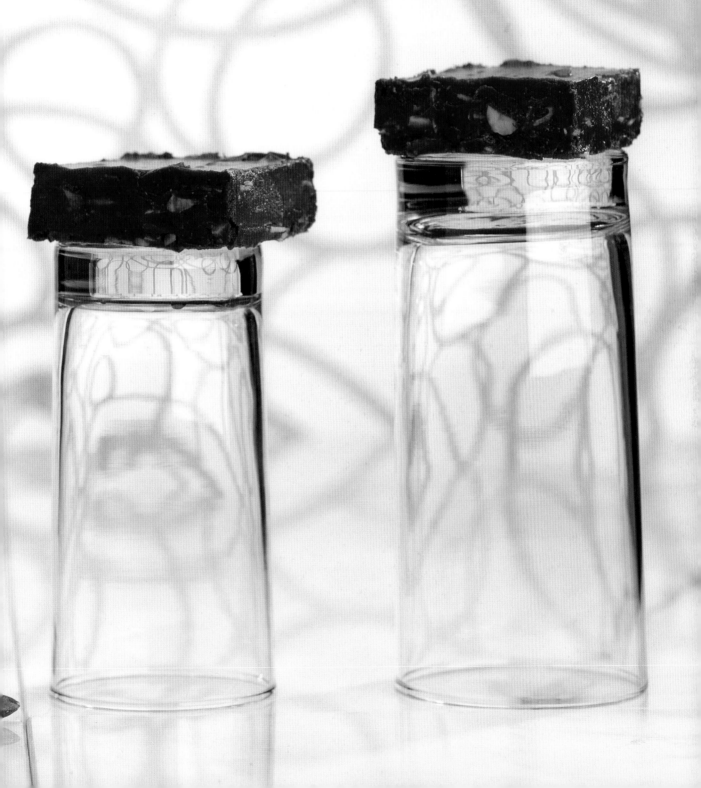

Spiced Nut Mix

Makes 4 cups (1 L)

3 Tbsp (45 mL) butter, melted

1 Tbsp (15 mL) garam masala

1 tsp (5 mL) ground ginger

⅛ tsp (0.5 mL) salt

1 cup (250 mL) pecan halves

1 cup (250 mL) walnut halves

1 cup (250 mL) whole almonds

½ cup (125 mL) cashews

½ cup (125 mL) peanuts

Preheat oven to 300° F (150° C). Combine butter, garam masala, ginger and salt in a large bowl. Add the nuts and toss until coated. Arrange in a single layer on a greased baking sheet with sides. Bake for about 20 minutes, stirring twice, until darkened and fragrant.

Ginger has been used both as a flavouring and medicinally for thousands of years. Not only does it add a nice warming flavour kick, but it also aids in digestion, has anti-inflammatory properties, helps boost circulation and lowers cholesterol and blood pressure. Ginger has also been credit with relieving headaches, treating arthritis pain and lowering fevers.

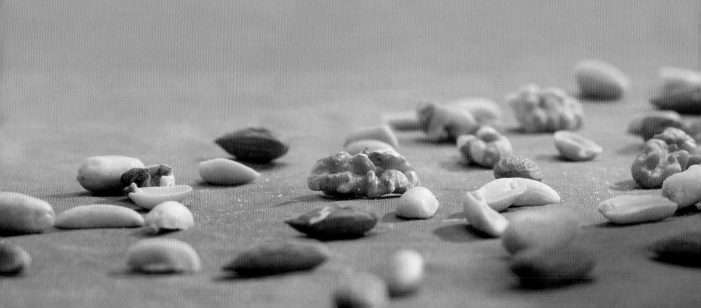

I had a little nut tree, nothing would it bear;
But a golden nutmeg and a silver pear.

—Mother Goose

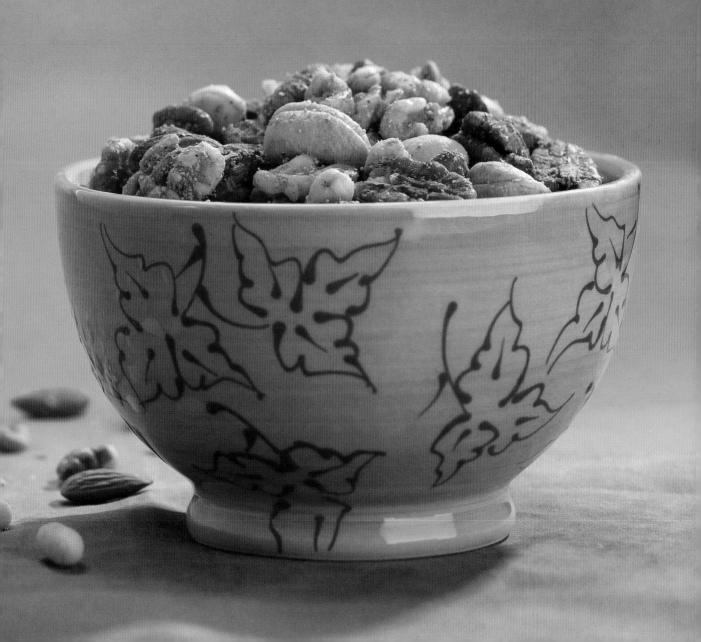

There Be Treasure in the Seas!

One Fish, Two Fish, Old Fish, New Fish

Rock paintings from all over the world depicting fish and innumerable remains of fossilized fish bones prove that humans have been finding Nemo since the dawn of time. The oldest known archeaological find of sea fish, at Terra Amata in Nice, France, is 380,000 years old. Humans must have quickly realized that the sea was a good way to satisfy their need for protein. Indeed, there are over 20,000 species of fish under the sea, most of them edible. It's likely that the world's first fishermen caught sluggish fish from the shallows of rivers by hand or grabbed those that were stranded on the seashore by the tide. It wouldn't have taken long to progress to fishing with spears and harpoons once the tools had been developed. All ancient human civilizations relied on fish, but at the top of the league for the consumption of fish and seafood, then as they are now, were the Japanese.

Made in Japan

In the West, the thought of eating raw fish was once considered taboo. However, during the past decade or so, sushi and sashimi have become not only acceptable, but also immeasurably popular. Japanese cuisine is considered healthy, tasty and nutritious. The Japanese have also popularized sea vegetables such as hijiki, wakame, kombu, nori and kanten. These seaweeds contain all the minerals found in the ocean and are excellent sources of iodine, iron, calcium, magnesium and vitamin K. Many sea vegetables contain sulfated polysaccharides called fucoidans that display potent anti-inflammatory activity by decreasing phospholipase A2, an enzyme that is important in the creation of the omega-6 fatty acid arachidonic acid. Fucoidans have also been studied for their antiviral activity and their benefits in reducing cardiovascular disease and colon cancer. Intake of sea vegetables also appears to modify estrogen cycles that can play a role in the risk of breast cancer. Seaweeds such as nori and hijiki are incredibly high in fibre and protein, and the latter probably has the most calcium of any sea green: 1400 mg per 100 g dry weight.

The Fat of the Sea

Fish have obtained their status as a superfood because of their high content of omega-3 fatty acids. Virtually nothing bad can be said about these healthy fats. There are two essential fats that we must get from our diet: omega-3 and omega-6 fatty acids. The omega-6 fats are not a problem because they're found in large amounts in vegetables, grain-fed meat, eggs and various vegetable oils. Getting adequate amounts of omega-3 fatty acids, on the other hand, seems to be much more difficult in our Western diet. Just a few thousand years ago, the ratio of omega-6 to omega-3 was close to 1:1. Today the ratio is closer to 20:1, an imbalance that has negative repercussions on our health regarding the development of cardiovascular disease and cancer. In general, our bodies use omega-6s to synthesize pro-inflammatory molecules, while omega-3s are used to synthesize anti-inflammatory ones. Because inflammation is a major factor in the development of chronic disease, nutritionists recommend that at least two serving of fatty fish be consumed every week to try to raise our intake of omega-3s.

Linolenic acid, an omega-3 fatty acid of plant origin, is found in large quantities in phytoplankton and is synthesized into longer chains of omega-3 fatty acids by fish. Two of these, eicosapentaenoic acid (EPA) and docosahexaenoic acid (DHA), make up a large part of our brain and the retina, and are critical in their development. They are also converted to hormones that affect our heart and immune function and, as mentioned earlier, reduce inflammation. We can convert linolenic acid to EPA and DHA, but the enzymes needed to do so are the same ones that convert omega-6s into pro-inflammatory compounds. So in a typical omega-6-rich Western diet, we are not efficient in synthesizing EPA and DHA. We are much better off obtaining pre-made EPA and DHA from animals that have already synthesized it from linolenic acid themselves. So eat the fish instead of the plankton; they're not only a better source of omega-3s, but they're easier to fry up.

Oh Me! Oh My! Omega Three!

The greatest nutritional deficiency affecting North America and Europe is a low intake of omega-3 fatty acids. These polyunsaturated fats are unstable and prone to oxidation, so try to obtain them from whole foods as much as possible rather than from supplements. Studies show that omega-3s are able to reduce the incidence of cardiovascular disease through several mechanisms. They reduce blood lipid levels, which in turn reduce the risk of plaque formation and atherosclerosis; they reduce the risk of cardiac arrhythmia, the most common cause of sudden death from cardiovascular illness; and they reduce the risk of inflammation of the cells that line blood vessels. Intake of omega-3s is also associated with a decrease in the incidence of certain cancers, namely colon, pancreatic, breast and prostate, by acting directly on the tumours and modifying their capacity to avoid cell death (apoptosis) and decreasing their blood supply. Their anti-inflammatory properties also help prevent the onset of cancer. The benefits of omega-3 fatty acids are many and varied, but these can only really be felt if the consumption of omega-6 fatty acids is reduced as well.

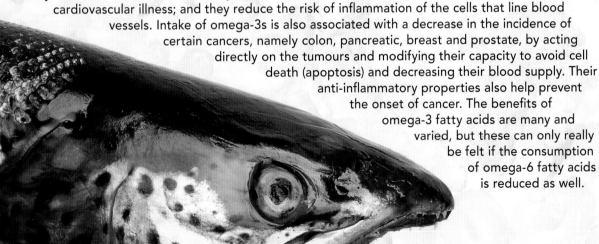

Salmon

Salmon is possibly the best source of omega-3 fatty acids on the planet. However, not all salmon are created equal. Because salmon has become such a popular food, salmon farming has become a huge industry. Farmed salmon are raised in high concentrations in aquatic pens, where they are fed grain instead of their natural diet of plankton, sardines and other species of fish. Also, because so many fish live in such close quarters, they are fed antibiotics to prevent the spread of disease. Choose wild salmon that feed naturally on plankton rather than hatchery salmon that are fed omega-6-rich grains. It may be a little bit more expensive, but it's well worth the health benefits.

Wild Salmon en Papillote

Serves 4

4 wild salmon fillets, 4 to 6 oz (115 to 170 g) each

4 leeks, white parts only, sliced thin and well washed

¼ cup (60 mL) dry white wine

sea salt and freshly ground pepper

1 bunch dill or other fresh herb, chopped

¼ cup (60 mL) unsalted butter, cut into 4 pieces

1 egg white, lightly beaten

1 lemon, sliced

a variety of sautéed vegetables

Heat oven to 350° F (175° C). Fold a 24 in (60 cm) sheet of parchment paper in half, and cut out a heart shape about 4 in (10 cm) larger than a fish fillet. Place fillet near fold, and place a handful of leeks next to it; sprinkle with wine, salt, pepper and dill and top with a piece of butter. Brush edges of parchment paper with egg white, fold paper to enclose fish, and make small overlapping folds to seal edges, starting at curve of heart. Be sure each fold overlaps previous one to create an airtight seal.

Repeat with rest of fillets. Put packages on a baking sheet, and bake until paper is puffed and brown, about 10 to 15 minutes. Serve salmon in packets with lemon slices and sautéed vegetables. Be careful of steam when opening packets.

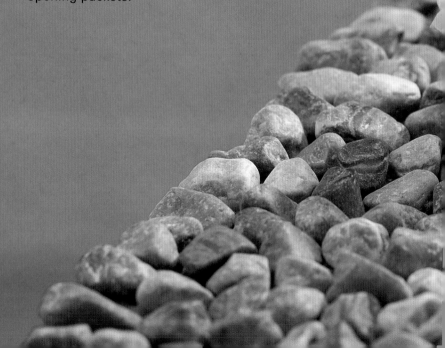

For the salmon dish on the cover, pan-fry or bake the fillets. Meanwhile, over medium, heat a splash of olive oil in a small pan. Saute 1 minced shallot and 1 Tbsp fresh thyme; add 1 cup blueberries, 1 cup water and 1 Tbsp balsamic vinegar. Reduce heat to low and simmer until sauce has reduced and thickened, about 6 minutes. Serve over salmon.

Fish is the best source of omega-3 fatty acids, yet concerns about environmental contamination with heavy metals has some people wondering if fish is safe to eat at all. Some fish species, especially those that are higher up on the food chain, do contain very small amounts of different toxic compounds, but it should be stressed that in such tiny quantities, the benefits obtained by eating fish far outweigh the risk. To be safe, limit your consumption of large predatory fish such as swordfish, shark and tuna to once a week, and eat salmon, sardines and mackerel twice or more per week.

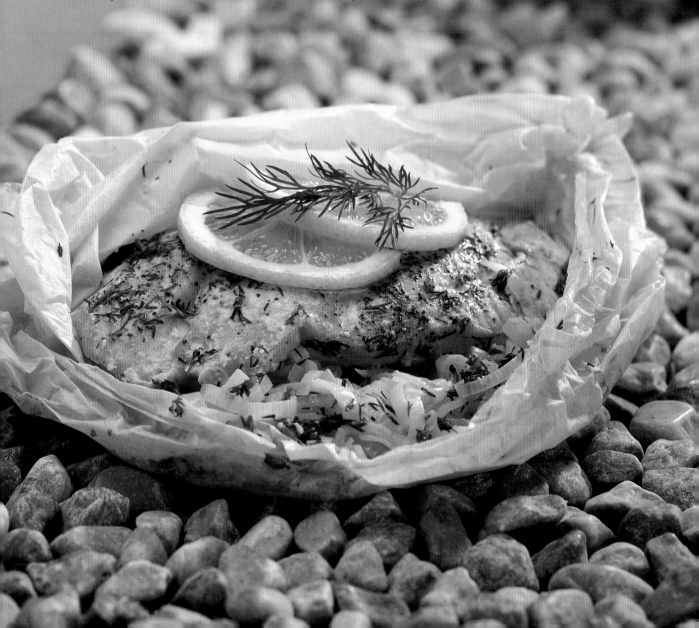

Sardines

Named after the Italian island of Sardinia, where they were once seen in huge schools, sardines are members of the herring family. They are small, silvery, soft-boned fish that feed primarily on plankton and are therefore not prone to the level of toxins that are found in predatory fish higher on the food chain. Sardines are loaded with protein, omega-3s and vitamin B12. They are also an excellent source of calcium as well as vitamin D, which helps increase the absorption of calcium and is therefore vital for maintaining healthy bones.

Baked Sardines with Gremolata

Serves 4

8 whole fresh sardines

sea salt and pepper

lemon wedges

canola oil as necessary

gremolata (see facing page)

Preheat oven to 350° F (175° C). Lightly oil a shallow baking dish just big enough to hold fish in a single layer. Sprinkle fish lightly on both sides with salt and pepper and lay in dish (skin side down if using fillets). Sprinkle half of gremolata on top of fish and drizzle with a little canola oil. Bake until cooked through, about 15 minutes. Transfer to serving plates, sprinkle with remaining gremolata and serve lemon wedge alongside.

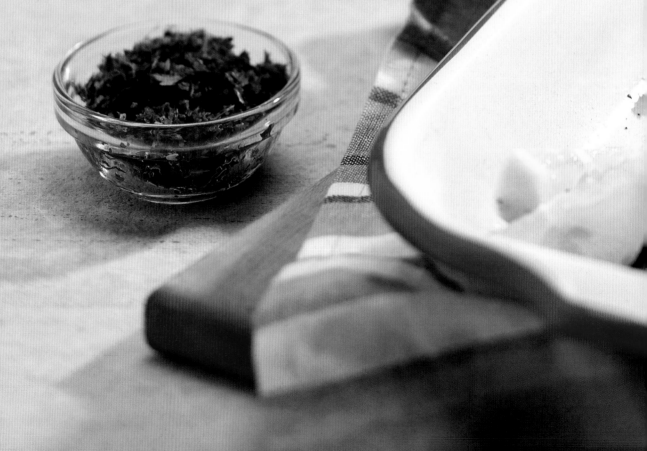

Combine parsley, garlic and lemon zest in a food processor. Pulse with an on/off motion until all ingredients are finely chopped and well combined. (Chopping can be done by hand if you don't have a food processor.)

Gremolata

½ cup (125 mL) flat-leaf parsley leaves

3 cloves garlic

zest of 1 lemon

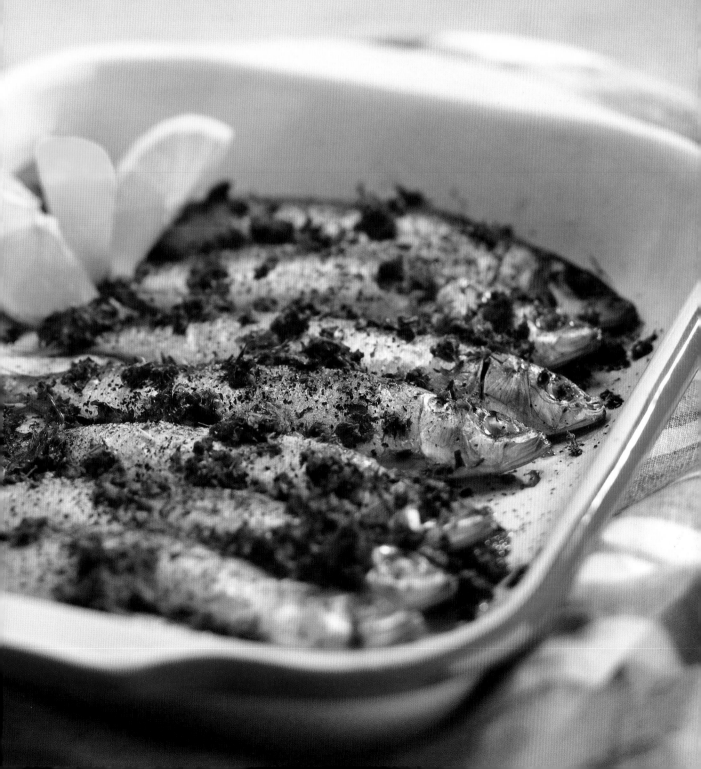

Wakame

Wakame, used traditionally to purify the blood and to give strength and luster to skin and hair, contains a compound known as fucoxanthin, which can burn fat. Japanese researchers have found that fucoxanthin induces the expression of the fat-burning protein UCP1 that accumulates in the fat that surrounds your internal organs. So the next time you take a seaweed bath to beautify your skin and hair, consider eating the stuff to lose weight, reduce inflammation and, while you're at it, get a healthy dose of all your ocean minerals.

Sesame Wakame Salad

Serves 4

$\frac{1}{3}$ **cup (80 mL) unseasoned rice vinegar**

1 Tbsp (15 mL) soy sauce

1 Tbsp (15 mL) agave nectar

6 Tbsp (90 mL) canola oil

2 Tbsp (30 mL) sesame oil

Combine rice vinegar, soy sauce and agave in a small bowl. Drizzle in both oils and whisk well.

(continued on next page)

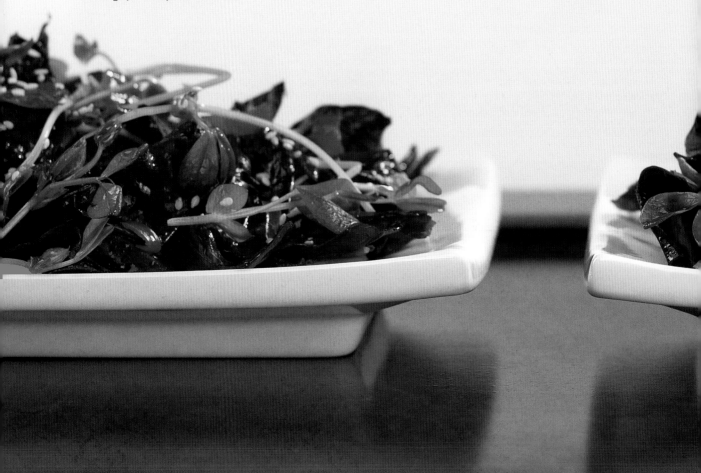

Place wakame in a large bowl. Add cold water to cover and set aside to soak for 3 to 5 minutes. Drain and squeeze out excess moisture. Cut into 4 in (10 cm) lengths. Place in a large bowl. Add sprouts. Drizzle dressing over, add chilis and toss to coat. Pile onto serving plates and sprinkle sesame seeds over top.

2 oz (55 g) dried wakame seaweed

1 cup (250 mL) loosely packed pea or radish sprouts

2 small red chili peppers, seeds and ribs removed, thinly sliced

¼ cup (60 mL) toasted sesame seeds

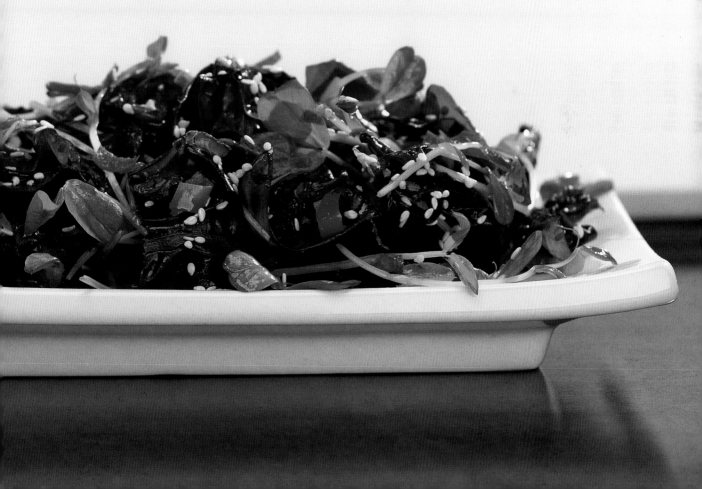

Nori

The term "nori" is used to refer to several types of seaweed from the *Porphyra* genus, a type of red algae that grows in the intertidal zone. *Porphyra* farming is big business in parts of Asia, particularly Japan and China; it is grown in the sea on nets that are suspended just below the surface of the water, and the farmers must tend to their crop by boat. Nori is available in the supermarket as thin dry sheets that look like blackish green paper; it is used extensively as a wrap for sushi but can also be thinly sliced and added to soups or ground and made into a paste. Nori is high in vitamin A and C, folate, riboflavin and potassium, and it is loaded with antioxidants, including carotenoids, and protein.

Nori Dip and Sauce

Makes ¼ cup (60 mL)

2 full sheets toasted nori, cut into thin strips

¼ cup (60 mL) water

1 Tbsp (15 mL) sake

1½ tsp (7 mL) soy sauce

½ tsp (2 mL) agave nectar

Place nori strips in a small saucepan. Add water, sake, soy sauce and agave nectar. Let sit until nori strips start to dissolve, 1 to 2 minutes. Stir together to form a paste. Place over low heat. Cook, stirring, until fragrant and smooth. Remove from heat and cool to room temperature. Once cool, transfer to a glass jar with a tight-fitting lid. Keep refrigerated for up to 2 weeks. Serve chilled or at room temperature as a dip for vegetables, or reheat to spread as a sauce over fish or roasted vegetables near end of their cooking time.

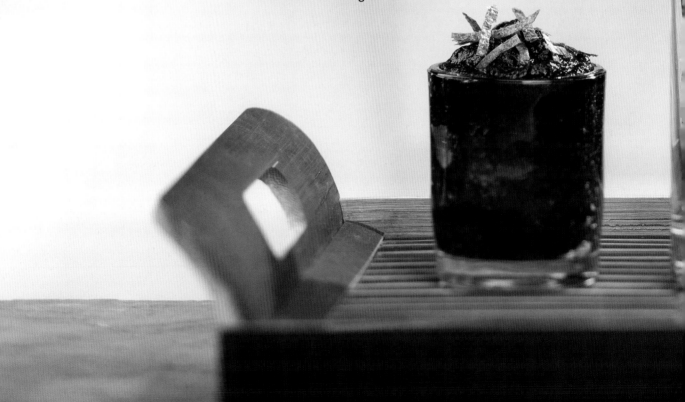

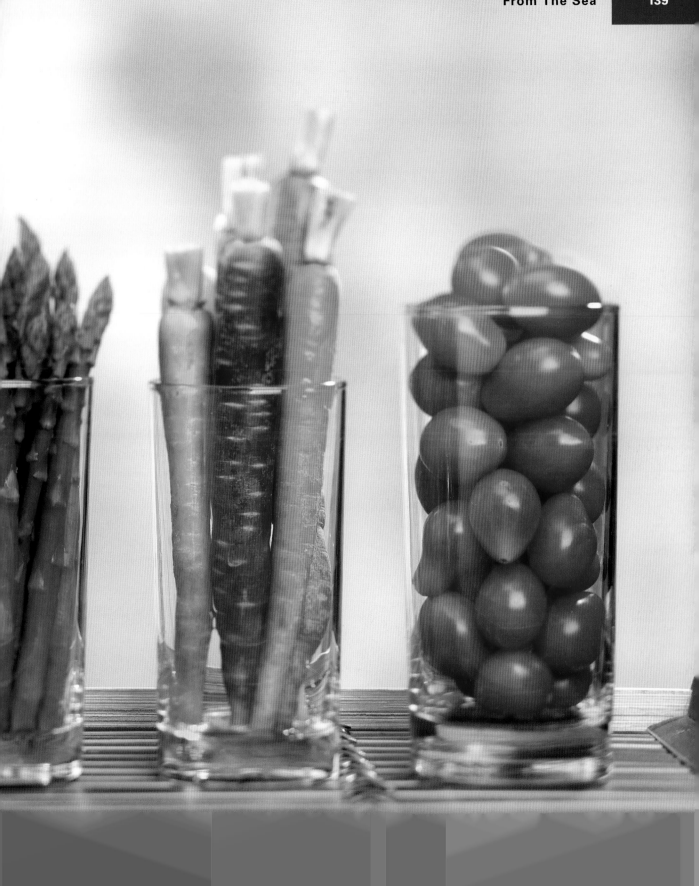

CHOCOLATE

Fruit of the Gods

It could be said that the Mayans were the world's first chocolate lovers, though the chocolate of their day bears little resemblance to the treat as we know it today. Chocolate is made from cacao beans, which grow on the cacao tree, whose scientific name *Theobroma cacao* is said to mean "fruit of the gods." To the Mayans, the cacao bean was sacred, and it featured heavily in their religion. They consumed their chocolate in liquid form; the cacao beans were ground and mixed with chilis and other spices, then added to hot water to make a spicy, somewhat bitter drink. The Aztecs also had a high opinion of the cacao bean. Like the Mayans, they too ground the beans and made them into a beverage, but for the Aztecs, the beans were not so easy to come by. Cacao trees are native to the Amazon Basin, quite a trek for the Aztecs. The beans were so prized by the Aztecs that they became a form of currency, and all taxes had to be paid in cacao beans.

Had he played his cards right, Christopher Columbus could have added "the man who introduced chocolate to Europe," to his list of credentials. However, because he failed to recognize the importance of the bean, even though he brought a few cacao plants back to Spain upon returning from the New World, the honour instead goes to Hernán Cortés, Spanish conquistador and overthrower of the Aztec Empire. In 1528, Cortés brought the beans to Spain's King Charles V and introduced him to the Aztec's cacao bean drink. However, Cortés had the clever idea of tossing a little sugar into the mixture, and the bitter beverage was transformed into a coveted delicacy. Within the next century or so, hot chocolate made its way throughout France and England, and eventually throughout most of Europe. As its popularity grew, so too did the number of ways that it was prepared, and by the 1840s, hot chocolate had been transformed yet again, this time into the solid chocolate bars that we know and love today.

Everything is Better with Chocolate

As children, we listened to our parents hound us about the importance of eating our veggies; perhaps they should have told us to eat our chocolate, as well. It's difficult to believe that something so decadent can also be good for us, but thankfully, it's true! Well, to a certain extent, anyway. In the production of chocolate, cacao beans are roasted, shelled and ground into a paste. The paste is then separated into cocoa solids and cocoa liquor. To make chocolate, the cocoa solids are mixed with cocoa butter and sugar; how much of each ingredient is used depends on what type of chocolate is being made—bitter, semi-sweet, milk, etc.

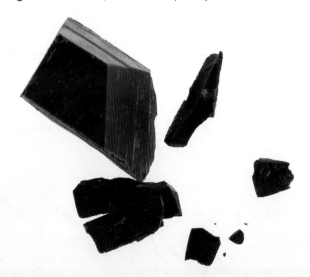

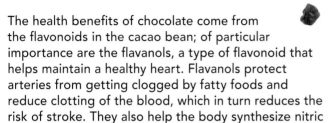

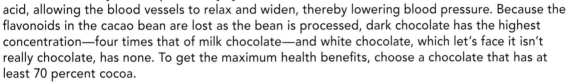

The health benefits of chocolate come from the flavonoids in the cacao bean; of particular importance are the flavanols, a type of flavonoid that helps maintain a healthy heart. Flavanols protect arteries from getting clogged by fatty foods and reduce clotting of the blood, which in turn reduces the risk of stroke. They also help the body synthesize nitric acid, allowing the blood vessels to relax and widen, thereby lowering blood pressure. Because the flavonoids in the cacao bean are lost as the bean is processed, dark chocolate has the highest concentration—four times that of milk chocolate—and white chocolate, which let's face it isn't really chocolate, has none. To get the maximum health benefits, choose a chocolate that has at least 70 percent cocoa.

Chocolate also contains theobromine, an antioxidant that helps lower blood pressure and has relaxing effects.

It is true that chocolate is a high fat food, the fat coming from the cocoa butter, but that is not necessarily bad news. Cocoa butter contains three types of fat: oleic acid, stearic acid and palmitic acid. Oleic acid is the type of fat found in olive oil and is a heart healthy, unsaturated fat. Stearic acid is a saturated fat, but research indicates that it has does not raise cholesterol level. There is nothing good to be said about palmitic acid, but at least it only makes up one-third of the total fat in cocoa butter.

Chocoholics Anonymous

Chocolate's status as a superfood does not mean that you have a free rein to indulge whenever the mood strikes. Chocolate is a high-fat, calorie-laden food, and overconsumption can lead to obesity, which has a wealth of negative health effects. Other foods, such as berries, pomegranate and red grapes are also excellent sources of flavonoids, but they are loaded with other essential nutrients as well. The key, as with all things in life, is moderation.

Raw Chocolate Mousse

Serves 4

½ cup (125 mL) pitted dates, soaked in boiling water for 20 minutes

6 Tbsp (90 mL) agave nectar

1 tsp (5 mL) vanilla

4 avocados

½ cup (125 mL) raw cacao powder

¼ cup (60 mL) coconut oil

¼ cup (60 mL) water

Combine dates, agave nectar and vanilla in a blender and purée until smooth. Add avocado, cacao powder and coconut oil and purée until smooth and creamy. Add only as much water as needed to thin to desired consistency, and purée until incorporated. Transfer to covered container and chill for at least 30 minutes before serving. Store in refrigerator for up to 3 days or in freezer up to 2 weeks.

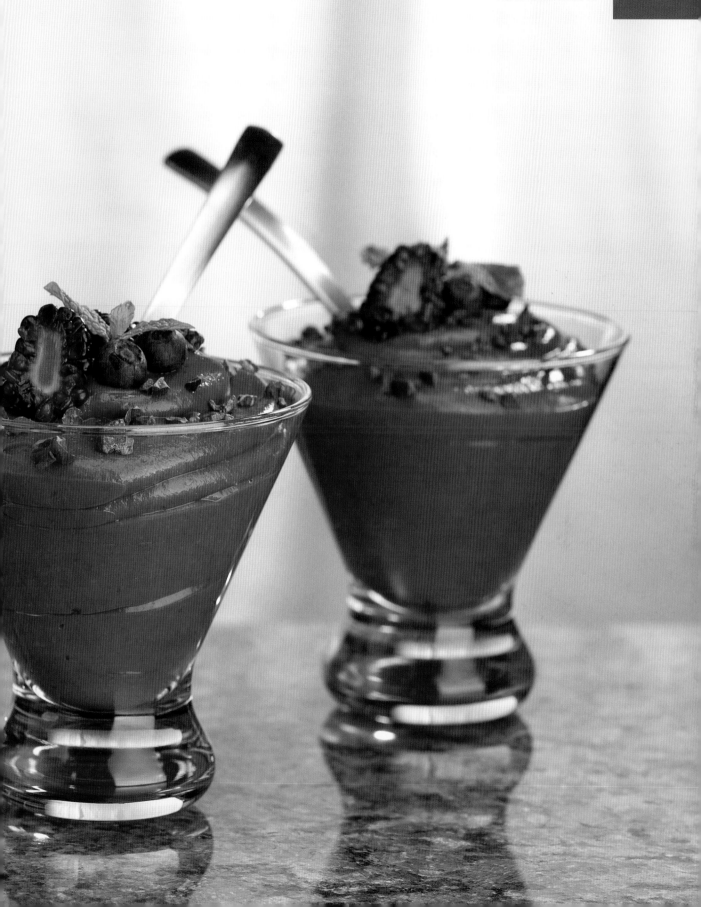

Raw Chocolate Hot Cocoa

Serves 4

½ cup (125 mL) hot water

1 Tbsp (15 mL) coconut oil

1 Tbsp (15 mL) raw honey

2 Tbsp (30 mL) cashew butter

5 Tbsp (75 mL) plus 2 tsp (10 mL) raw cacao powder

1 tsp (5 mL) vanilla

pinch of sea salt

pinch of cayenne or chili powder, optional

2½ cups (625 mL) soy or almond milk, warmed

Combine hot water, coconut oil, honey, cashew butter, cacao powder, vanilla, salt and chili powder or cayenne (if using) in a blender and purée until smooth. (Can be done ahead up to this point and kept covered in refrigerator for up to 5 days.) Divide among 4 mugs and stir in warm soy or almond milk.

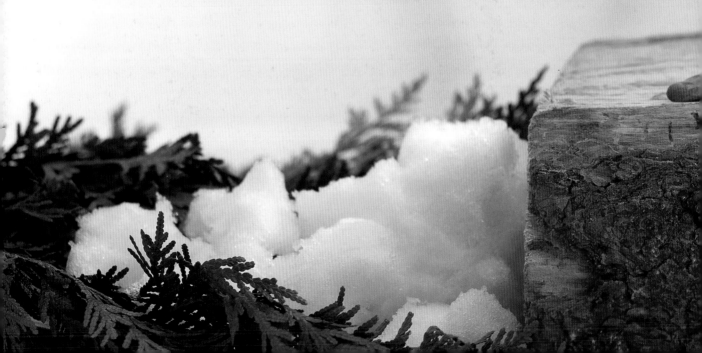

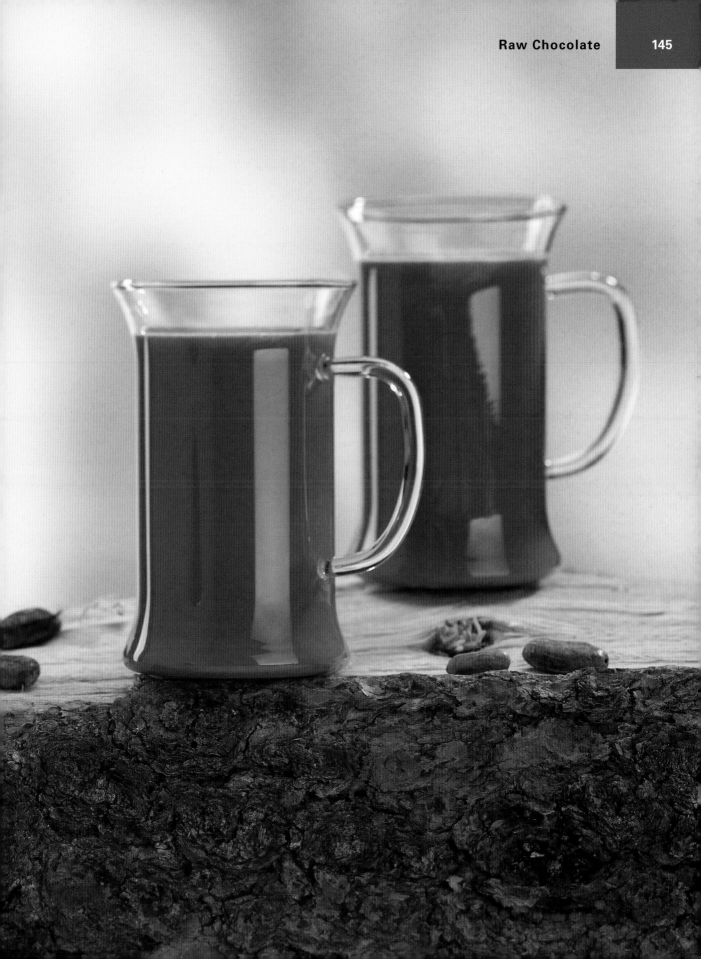

THE GOOD GUT BUGS

Food of the Centenarians

Bulgaria proudly claims to be a country with one of the highest number of people who live to be 100 and over. Their secret to long life is a frugal diet consisting mainly of yogurt, a fermented milk product that the Balkan country claims to have invented. Bulgarian yogurt is not curdled milk but the product of two lactic bacteria acting together. *Lactobacillus bulgaricus* makes lactic acid from lactose, the sugar found in milk, and *Streptococcus thermophylus* provides the characteristic aroma. The probiotic bacteria used to make kefir include some types that are not found in yogurt, such as *Lactobacillus caucasus* and *Leuconostoc* and *Acetobacter* species. The kefir of the Balkans, Eastern Europe and the Caucus is made from the addition of kefir granules—a complex combination of bacteria, yeasts, proteins, sugars and lipids—to cow, sheep or goat's milk. The end product is a fizzy drink that is both acidic and slightly alcoholic, sometimes up to a strength of 2% alcohol. The lactic acid produced in yogurt and kefir may not guarantee a sure path to becoming a centenarian, but its effects on the digestive system are excellent. It creates an acidic environment in the gut that destroys unfriendly bacteria that cause putrefaction, a term that is the direct opposite of digestion. Putrefaction is just as unpleasant as it sounds.

Bulgarian yogurt was introduced to Western Europe as early as 1542, when French King Francis I was suffering from severe depression. The doctors could do nothing for his listlessness and apathy until he was told of a Turkish doctor who made a brew of fermented sheep's milk, which people spoke of in glowing terms. The king sent for the doctor, who refused to travel except on foot, along with his entire flock of sheep. After a very long walk through southern Europe, the doctor finally arrived and put the king (now irate and impatient) on a regime of sheep's milk yogurt for several weeks. The king was cured at last and invited the doctor to stay in his court. Unfortunately, the sheep couldn't fully recover from their long trip or adjust to the Parisian climate; after the last animal died, the doctor left Paris, taking with his the secret of his medicinal brew. And yogurt was forgotten for nearly four centuries.

The Legen-dairy Probiotics

Although Bulgarians may have instinctively known that their yogurt was the fountain of youth, it wasn't until the early 1900s that Russian scientist Ilya Mechnikov, a 1908 Nobel Prize winner, linked yogurt with longevity. Later, scientists in Europe, Japan and the U.S. proved the bacteria in yogurt helped maintain good health by protecting us from toxins, infections, allergies and some types of cancer.

The fermentation process can render foods that were previously inedible and even dangerous into something tasty and somewhat nutritious. In grains, lectins, gluten and phytates can be vastly reduced by fermentation. Rejuvelac is a fermented drink prepared by sprouting a grain and then soaking it in water for a few days, and consuming the liquid. Fermentation also breaks down the lactose in milk, thus mitigating a problem for those who are lactose intolerant or those on a low-carb diet. The greatest benefit of fermentation, however, is the introduction of helpful probiotic bacteria to our guts. These microorganisms improve digestion and promote gut health, which means we can absorb more nutrients, vitamins and minerals. This is particularly relevant for those who eat plenty of phytate-rich foods that bind minerals and render them unavailable. Probiotics restore the balance of our intestinal flora to one that inhibits the growth of pathogenic and toxin-producing bacteria. They alleviate chronic intestinal inflammatory diseases such as irritable bowel syndrome, Crohn's disease and colitis. Clinical trials are mixed, but several small studies show that certain probiotics may help maintain remission of ulcerative colitis and prevent the relapse of Crohn's disease. More research is needed to determine which strain works best for which condition. For irritable bowel syndrome, *Bifidobacterium animalis, B. infantis* and *Lactobacillus plantarum* seem effective, while *L. acidophilus* reduces intestinal inflammation and the size of intestinal tumours.

Probiotics are also useful in maintaining urogenital health. The vagina, like the intestines, needs a finely balanced ecosystem. The dominant *Lactobacilli* strain usually make it too acidic for harmful bacteria to take hold. Any number of factors, including antibiotics and birth control pills, can upset this balance and cause bacterial vaginosis, yeast infection and urinary tract infection. Probiotics help restore the pH balance and prevent or treat these urogenital problems.

The best case for probiotic therapy has been for the treatment of diarrhea. Taking antibiotics to treat an infection or illness may alter the microflora and their metabolism of carbohydrates. Bacteria are able to absorb short-chain fatty acids that result from carb metabolism, but when their numbers are reduced as a result of antibiotics, these fatty acids cause an osmotic upset that results in diarrhea. Another potential consequence of taking antibiotics is the opportunistic overgrowth of pathogenic organisms like *Clostridium difficile.* Although studies are limited and sometimes inconsistent, two large reviews suggest that probiotics reduce antibiotic-associated diarrhea by 60%, when compared with a placebo.

Go Forth and Ferment Thy Food

Before there were hand sanitizers, before there were refrigerators, and even before we even knew about the existence of microorganisms, humans likely ate a rotting fruit or an old carcass from time to time. It's possible that we evolved to handle a little microorganism in our food because of the seamless integration of bacteria into our lives. Only later did we start fermenting our food on purpose, and we've been doing so ever since. Once the existence of microorganisms was discovered in the 1600s, it took a few more centuries to figure out that they caused disease. As usual, we went overboard and declared an all-out war on germs. We pasteurize, sanitize, irradiate and clean everything around us in our irrational, seemingly innate fear of these tiny invisible organisms. Paying attention to cleanliness and hygiene is inarguably important, but in the case of fermented foods, the more germ-ridden the food, the better.

COCONUT KEFIR

Kefir can be made from both dairy and non-dairy sources. For a non-dairy beverage, the kefir granules can be added to soymilk, rice milk or coconut water. Coconut water kefir is virtually non-allergenic and helps sooth a number of digestive issues including flatulence, bloating and *Candida* overgrowth. Coconut water is also an excellent source of potassium, which helps lower the risk of high blood pressure, provides intracellular hydration and supports the proper functioning of muscle and nerve cells.

To make coconut kefir, pour 4 cups (1 L) of room temperature coconut water (from two to three green coconuts, see Tip, p. 12) into a lidded container large enough to leave some space for air. Stir in a kefir starter packet. For a fizzy kefir, seal the container tightly; for a non-fizzy one, cover the container but do not seal it. Let the mixture sit at room temperature for 24 to 48 hours, depending on the temperature. Your kefir is ready when it turns a milky colour and tastes tangy and tart rather than sweet; there will usually be a little foam on top. Keep it in the refrigerator for up to two weeks. You can drink the kefir plain, with a twist of lime or mixed with an equal amount of unsweetened fruit juice.

When you're ready to make more kefir, stir $\frac{1}{4}$ cup (60 mL) of your last batch into 4 cups (1 L) fresh coconut water and ferment as above. In this way, seven batches of kefir can be made from one packet of starter.

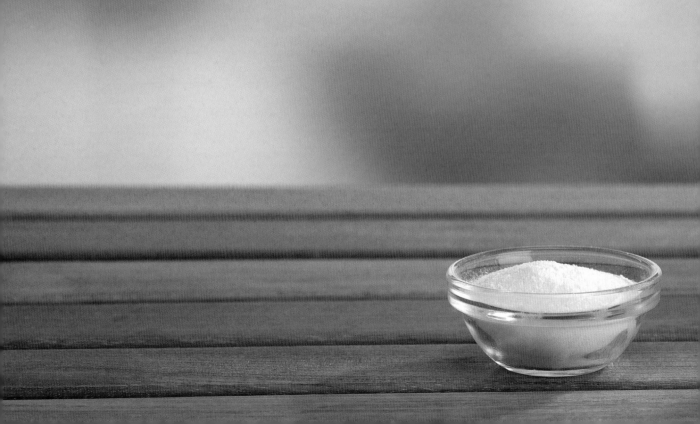

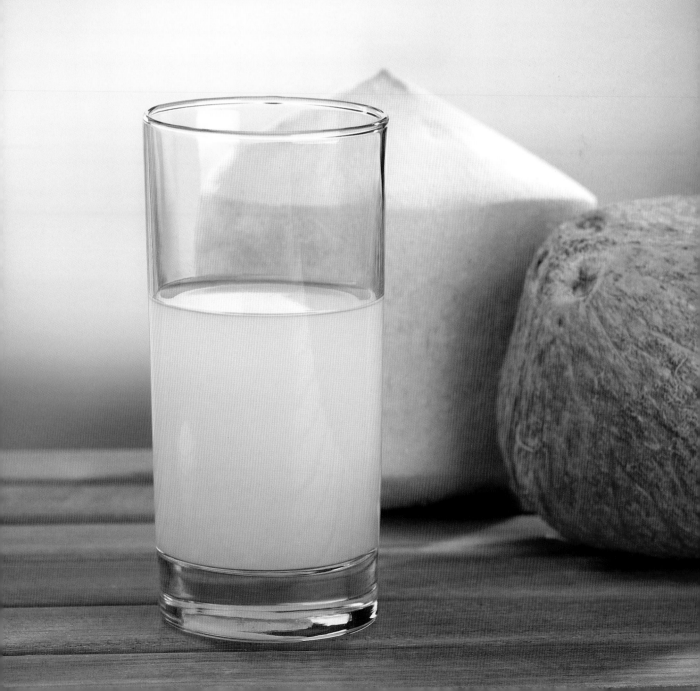

Though the term "fermented" sounds vaguely distasteful, the results of this ancient preparation and preservation technique—produced through the breakdown of carbohydrates and proteins by microorganisms such as bacteria, yeasts and molds—are actually delicious.

—Dr. Mercola

REJUVELAC

Rejuvelac can be made from whole wheat, rye, quinoa, oats, barley, millet, buckwheat or rice, but rye and wheat seem to be the tastiest. To begin, make sure all vessels and utensils are spotlessly clean. Place 1/2 cup (125 mL) of wheat or rye berries in a 6 cup (1.5 L) or larger glass jar. Cover with at least 2 cups (500 mL) of cool (60 to 70° F [16 to 21° C]) filtered water. Cover the mouth of the jar with a piece of screen or cheese cloth (to keep any bugs or dust from landing in it) and secure with an elastic band. Let it stand 8 hours or overnight.

Drain the water from the jar. Rinse the wheat (or rye) berries with cool filtered water and drain again. Keep the jar covered as above. Prop the bottom end of the jar up at a 45-degree angle to drain any excess water. Allow 24 to 48 hours for the wheat berries to sprout, rinsing and draining 3 times at regular intervals each day. The sprouts are ready when the tails are 1/4 in (0.5 cm) long.

Rinse and drain the sprouts one last time. Add 4 cups (1 L) of cool filtered water. Let the mixture stand, still covered with a screen, at room temperature (at least 70° F [21° C]) out of direct light for between 12 and 48 hours, depending on the temperature, to ferment. Stir gently once each day while it ferments. The mixture should be slightly cloudy and milky and may have some foam on top. It should taste sour, but not spoiled. Strain the liquid into a second sterilized glass jar. This is rejuvelac. Screw a lid on tightly over the rejuvelac and store in the refrigerator for up to 5 days.

The same sprouts can be used to make 2 more batches of rejuvelac. Once the first batch of rejuvelac has been strained off, do not rinse the sprouts. Add 4 cups (1 L) of filtered water to the jar and let stand another 12 to 48 hours. Second and third batches will ferment faster than the first, so check the rejuvelac sooner and more often. After the third batch, the sprouted wheat should be discarded.

You can drink rejuvelac by itself, chilled or at room temperature, or try blending 1 cup (250 mL) with 1/2 cup (125 mL) of fresh strawberries or other fruit until smooth.

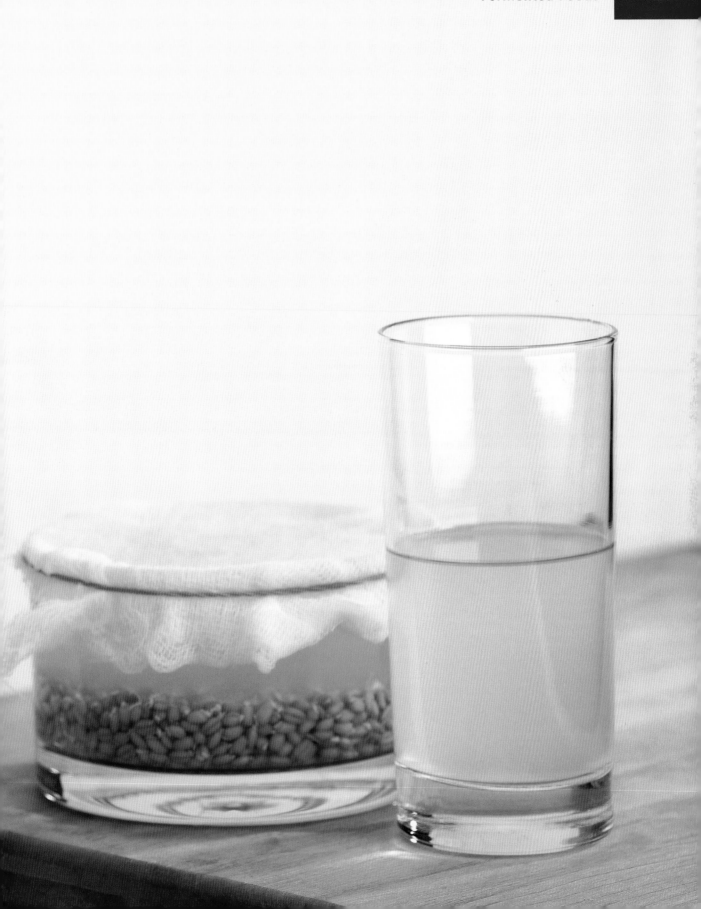

JUST YOUR CUP OF TEA

A Spot of Tea

During World War II's D-Day, the plan was to advance until nightfall to capture as much ground as possible before the expected German counter attack. American troops were upset over reports that the British troops had stopped advancing to make tea. The British had in fact started brewing their tea as soon as they landed on Sword Beach, even though they were under heavy fire. This story goes to show how important tea was to the British. During the war, more tea was shipped to the troops than anything except small arms ammunition. One soldier observed that they were damn lucky the Germans never tried baiting minefields with tea.

The tea plant, *Camilla sinensis,* originated in China and has risen to the status of the second most popular drink in the world. The first is water. Every second, 15,000 cups of tea are being consumed on the planet. According to Chinese legend, tea was discovered around 5000 BC by emperor Shen Nong, who was boiling some water in his garden when some leaves fell in and he decided to taste the fragrant brew.

Black, Green and In Between

Black, green and oolong tea all come from the same plant, but the fermentation process produces an end result that gives each one a completely different chemical composition. Green tea is the least transformed and contains the most antioxidant polyphenols. Black tea is roasted and rolled before fermentation, which converts the polyphenols into black pigments. Oolong is a semi-fermented tea that puts its flavour and properties somewhere between green and black.

Green Tea EGCG, Find Out What it Means to Me

Most of the research on green tea has focused on its anticancer activity. Green tea's most abundant polyphenol, epigallocatechin gallate (EGCG), may be useful in the prevention of leukemia and renal, bladder, skin, breast, mouth, stomach, pancreatic and prostate cancers, and it may decrease the severity of the initial diagnosis and the likelihood of recurrence. EGCG is also one of the most powerful dietary compounds that can inhibit angiogenesis, the process involving the formation of new blood vessels needed for a tumour to grow.

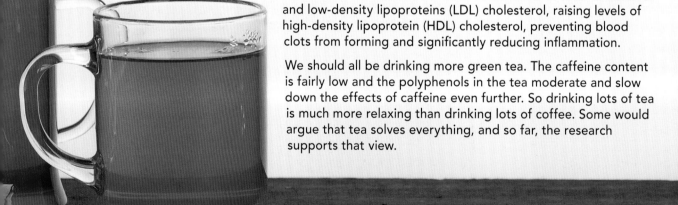

Green tea and EGCG also reduce blood levels of total cholesterol and low-density lipoproteins (LDL) cholesterol, raising levels of high-density lipoprotein (HDL) cholesterol, preventing blood clots from forming and significantly reducing inflammation.

We should all be drinking more green tea. The caffeine content is fairly low and the polyphenols in the tea moderate and slow down the effects of caffeine even further. So drinking lots of tea is much more relaxing than drinking lots of coffee. Some would argue that tea solves everything, and so far, the research supports that view.

IN VINO VERITAS

Age Before Beauty

Considering the immense importance of wine to human civilization, it is not surprising that it has always been regarded as having medicinal properties. Hippocrates, the founder of modern medicine, often prescribed wine to treat all manner of ailments. Pliny the Elder, author of the voluminous *Naturalis Historia,* wrote: "Wine alone of itself is a remedy; it nourishes the blood, pleases the stomach and calms worry and care." And it seems as though the ancients had it right. Wine, in moderation, is good for us.

The first glimpse of evidence came to be known as the "French Paradox." Researchers wondered why the French had an unusually low mortality rate from heart disease despite a lifestyle that included high rates of smoking and a diet rich in saturated fats and cholesterol. Wine consumption emerged as a protective factor, and future studies confirmed this finding, but only for moderate consumption of two to four glasses for men and one to two glasses for women per day. Anything over these amounts and the health benefits not only disappear, but the mortality risks increases rapidly.

Resveratrol Is in the House Wine

Wine reduces the risk of cardiovascular disease by causing an increase in high-density lipoprotein (HDL) and a decrease in the tendency of blood to form clots. It contains myriad polyphenols that occur predominantly in the skins and seeds of grapes, including resveratrol, a plant hormone that may be responsible red wine's health benefits.

Resveratrol is produced whenever the grape plant is under environmental stress, which means that the soil type, slope, climate, humidity, presence of fungus, predators, microorganisms, insects and other stressors will affect its expression. The cardiovascular protective effects of resveratrol may offer a form of preconditioning rather than direct therapy, meaning that drinking wine may prevent as well as treat heart disease.

Resveratrol also ameliorates diabetes symptoms, reduces inflammation, inhibits the growth of some viruses, protects the brain and nervous system and lowers the risk of developing Alzheimer's. In 1996, it was identified as the first molecule of dietary origin capable of interfering with all thee stages of cancer development: initiation, promotion and progression. Resveratrol can also activate a family of proteins known as sirtuins, which repair DNA as cells age and extend cell life.

Dine on Wine

Obtaining resveratrol from red wine is one of the best ways to receive its health benefits. The resveratrol sold as nutritional supplements is produced by biotechnical synthesis and is derived from Japanese knotweed. Although resveratrol pills can deliver a large dose at once, bioavailability is extremely low. Resveratrol doesn't dissolve well in water, which is why the alcohol content of wine helps its delivery into our bodies. If you don't drink alcohol, you can get resveratrol from other sources such as red grapes, grape juice, peanuts and pomegranates. If you already drink, drink moderately, raise your glass, and say cheers to your good health.

No Such Thing as Too Much Garlic

Everyone Loves Garlic (except Vampires)

French Chef Philippe Gion recounts the story of Anibal Comous, a Marseillais who lived to be 104 and maintained that he kept his youth and brilliance by eating garlic every day. When his 80-year-old son died, the father mourned: "I always told him he wouldn't live long, poor boy. He ate too little garlic!"

Garlic is one of the oldest plants to be used as a medicine and is the world's most commonly used flavouring. Ancient cultures developing in isolation from one another came to many of the same conclusions about garlic's action and efficacy. The earliest known reference for garlic's medicinal use is the *Codex Ebers*, an ancient Egyptian text dating from 1500 BC that prescribes the bulb for circulatory ailments, general malaise and infestation with insects and parasites. Research would later confirm its effectiveness in reducing cardiovascular disease, and as a potent antibacterial, antiviral and antifungal agent.

There is evidence that in ancient Greece garlic was fed to soldiers going off to battle and to athletes during the earliest Olympics, making it perhaps the world's first performance-enhancing drug. In ancient Rome, Pliny the Elder (23–79 AD), a Greek physician, listed no less than 61 garlic-based cures in his five-volume *Historica Naturalis*. In ancient China, garlic was in wide use since before 2000 BC; it formed part of the daily diet, was prescribed for respiratory ailments and digestion, and was used in combination therapy to treat fatigue, headache and insomnia. During the Middle Ages garlic was used extensively to treat the plague, and much later, during the 1700s, against scurvy and asthma. It wasn't until 1858 that a definitive demonstration of garlic's potent antibacterial properties was made by Louis Pasteur. The folklore surrounding garlic and onions worldwide is vast, but recent studies have found that these plants have more serious health benefits for the heart and cancer prevention than folklore could ever have predicted.

May the Stink be With You

Garlic, onions, leeks, shallots and chives all belong to the *Allium* genus. They are odourless when fresh, but as soon as they are crushed or cut, a chemical change occurs resulting in their characteristic pungent flavour and aroma. The compounds responsible contain sulphur, securing members of this genus a place in the smelly food club (along with cruciferous vegetables). When you cut an onion, propanethial S-oxide is released and causes your eyes to flow like Niagara Falls. To avoid the tears, rinse the peeled bulb under a running tap because the compound is water-soluble. When you cut, crush or chew garlic, the compound alliin is enzymatically converted to allicin, a very strong-smelling molecule that is directly responsible for the way garlic tastes. The gaseous metabolite allyl methyl sulfide is what causes "garlic breath." It is absorbed into the blood during metabolism, travels to the lungs, and from there, to the mouth and into the face of your neighbour. The gas is also exuded through your skin pores, and washing with soap and water doesn't seem to help. Drinking milk with garlic (not after) reduces the odour because the mix of water and fat effectively binds the gas. Less effective, but much more appetizing, is combining water, basil and mushrooms with garlic.

Allium, MD

Almost everyone has heard of allicin thanks to manufacturers of garlic supplements, who base their claims of efficacy on high allicin content. The compound is highly unstable, however, raising doubts in some scientists as to the efficiency of its absorption and its biological activity. Allicin breaks down into a number of different sulphur-containing compounds such as ajoene, diallyl sulfide (DAS) and diallyl disulfide (DADS), each possessing interesting bioactivity on their own. Ajoene, applied topically, has been studied as an effective treatment for skin cancer. Both DAS and DADS are lipid-soluble and are considered to be the principle agents responsible for preventing the onset or the progression of stomach and esophageal cancer, and likely lung, breast and colon cancers as well. Other research has found that increasing garlic intake reduces carcinogenic nitrite levels in the body, resulting in fewer deaths from stomach cancer. Indeed, countries where garlic is consumed in higher amounts thanks to traditional cuisines have an overall lower incidence of cancer.

For cardiovascular health, garlic provides a multi-pronged assault on heart disease. In several studies, garlic supplementation reduced the accumulation of cholesterol in vascular walls, aortic plaques deposits, platelet aggregation and vascular calcification in patients with high blood cholesterol. Garlic's anticoagulant activity is useful in preventing clot formation but can also be dangerous if mixed with other blood-thinning medications, including aspirin. The metabolite hydrogen sulfide derived from the catabolism of garlic compounds in red blood cells causes blood vessels to dilate, thereby reducing the risk of hypertension. Garlic is a good source of vitamin C and other antioxidants that can significantly reduce the blood concentration of free radicals in patients with atherosclerosis, and prevent the oxidation of low-density lipoproteins, a key step in the initiation of blood plaques. Its selenium content also provides protection against oxidative stress because it is a crucial cofactor for the body's most important endogenous antioxidant, glutathione peroxidase. Garlic's vitamin B6 content also helps prevent heart disease by lowering levels of homocysteine, an intermediate product of the methylation cycle that can directly damage blood vessels.

All members of the *Allium* group contain compounds that inhibit enzymes involved in inflammation, making them useful in the treatment of inflammatory disorders such as asthma, osteoarthritis and rheumatoid arthritis.

Given garlic's plethora of health benefits, there is no doubt that it and other members of the Allium family deserve a place in your arsenal of disease-fighting superfoods. However, their medicinal and nutritional benefits are substantially reduced when they are in flake, powder or paste form: fresh is best. Choose garlic bulbs and onions that are clean, plump and have crisp, unbroken outer skin. If they are soft, shriveled, mouldy or have begun to sprout, don't eat them.

SUPPLEMENTS

Eating the Extra Edge

No matter how much we strive to maintain a healthy lifestyle or eat right, a number of obstacles in our modern world can easily thwart us. Artificial light seduces us into staying up later at night than we should. The Internet and other forms of electronic entertainment compete for our time when we should be outside taking in the sun and being active. Sometimes we don't have access to healthy foods. Supplementation may be that extra insurance we need to be our optimal selves in the 21st century. The natural health supplement industry is huge, and there are tons of products out there, some of them useful, and some of them useless. Be critical of the hype and try to see through the smoke of false or exaggerated health claims. That said, there are many supplements that can provide measurable health benefits, and there are others that have shown great promise. Here are a few superfoods that might just be the extra edge you need to be a modern day superhuman.

Psyllium: Fun with Fibre

Psyllium is a rather new supplement that has found its way into our breakfast cereals and other foods. The plant belongs to the genus *Plantago*, a native of Iran and India and a relative of our garden weed plantain. The tiny seeds are covered in a husk containing indigestible fibres that are soluble in water. The glycosides and mucilages in the husk cause it to swell up to 10 times its original volume when mixed with water. The soluble fibre is not broken down in our gut and has no nutritive value. When swelled with water, psyllium fibre stimulates the intestines to contract and help speed the passage of stool through the digestive tract. Because of its ability to soak up a significant amount of water, it can be used to treat mild diarrhea. Softer stools from fibre intake can also decrease the pain associated with hemorrhoids. Although fibre can help people with ulcerative colitis avoid remission, some people with inflammatory bowel disease have experienced a worsening of symptoms with psyllium supplementation. Psyllium also plays a role in lowering blood cholesterol. The fibre binds bile acids in the intestines, thus lowering cholesterol levels in the blood; however, it is only truly effective when combined with a diet low in saturated fat and cholesterol.

Psyllium is definitely a great source of fibre, but it's important to get fibre from all sources, including fruits, vegetables and legumes, which provide vitamins, minerals and a variety of beneficial phytochemicals. If you decide to supplement with psyllium fibre, gradually increase intake and drink 6 to 8 glasses of water per day to avoid possible gastrointestinal problems.

Spirulina: Food of the Future

During the Spanish exploration of South America, one of Cortés' soldiers described a "new food" being harvested from Lake Texcoco and sold as blue-green "cakes." The Aztecs called it *techuitlatl*, which means "stone's excrement," a pleasant-sounding food that has now become famous for its use by NASA as a dietary supplement for astronauts on space missions. Spirulina is a microscopic, thread-like blue-green algae (species *Arthrospina platensis* and *Arthrospir maxima*) that is rich in protein (up to 70% of its dry weight), vitamins, especially B12 and pro-vitamin A (beta-carotene), and minerals, especially iron. It is also rich in antioxidant phenolic acids, tocopherols and the omega-3 fatty acid, linolenic acid. Gram for gram, spirulina can contain 290% more calcium than whole milk and 8000% more iron than spinach. Spirulina is no doubt a nutritional powerhouse deserving of the title superfood, but the environmental cost associated with producing dried algae powder is significant: all single cell organisms contain mostly water, and it takes a lot of heat to produce a sizeable amount of powder. Also, because algae grow in water, they can easily become contaminated with pollutants, so make sure to get a high-quality supplement.

A well-documented benefit of spirulina is its ability to fight allergies; it inhibits the release of histamine and also exhibits anti-inflammatory properties. Research also shows that taking spirulina could reduce precancerous lesions in the mouth and reduce the risk of mouth cancer; reduce total cholesterol and low-density lipoprotein levels in healthy volunteers and those who have ischemic heart disease; and potentially act as an antiviral agent against herpes, influenza and HIV, and as a treatment for liver damage and cirrhosis.

Spirulina was promoted as "the best food for the future" by the United Nations World Food Conference in 1974. Several member states of the UN have formed the Intergovernmental Institution for the use of Micro-algae Spirulina Against Malnutrition (IIMSAM) who, along with scientists, aid organizations and African leaders, plan to make spirulina a key driver to eradicate malnutrition and achieve food security. Africa is ideal for spirulina. It grows naturally in lakes in Central Africa and has been used for centuries in Chad. From fighting world hunger to feeding space explorers, spirulina may truly be our number one superfood.

Mow Down the Wheatgrass

In his attempts to save his sick hens, Charles F. Schnabel fed them fresh cut grass. They not only recovered but they produced more eggs than usual. He repeated the experiment the following year and found that hens consuming rations supplemented with wheatgrass doubled their egg production. This was in 1931, and three years later, he applied for a patent for processing young wheat, barley and rye grass as a health food supplement for both animals and humans. Schnabel's research showed that the nutritional value of grasses peaked at the jointing stage, a period in the plant's life stage in which the concentrations of chlorophyll, protein and vitamins are at their highest. By 1940, cans of Schnabel's powdered grass were on sale in drugstores throughout North America. In the late 1960s, Anna Wigmore, a Lithuanian-born American whole foods advocate, developed the wheatgrass diet and made unsubstantiated health claims that it could eliminate the need for insulin in diabetics and cure AIDS. Don't believe all the hype you read about wheatgrass—the claims for its curative powers are bottomless. Know, however, that it is indeed very nutritious, healthy, and part of the superfoods family.

The active ingredient in wheatgrass is chlorophyll, the photosynthetic apparatus of all plants that gives them their green colour. There is some evidence that chlorophyll lowers rates of colon cancer, and it may be therapeutic for ulcerative colitis. Claims that wheatgrass helps blood flow and detoxification may have some credence as well. Wheatgrass can also bind toxic heavy metals and thus has a chelation effect. It probably isn't the miracle cure that some proponents make it out to be, but its concentrated nutrition makes it a fine addition to your juices and smoothies. You can buy it planted in trays, in capsules, liquid extracts, tinctures and juices, but perhaps the most rewarding way is to grow your own from seeds. Why not develop a grassy green thumb while you're enjoying your grassy green juice?

Index

About the Authors

Jennifer Sayers is a chef and writer who has been cooking professionally for nearly 20 years—although she started in the kitchen long before that. She is passionate about fresh, local ingredients and believes that cooking and eating with the seasons enhances our enjoyment of food.

Dr. Patrick Owen has a PhD in Human Nutrition from McGill University, and he uses his expertise in traditional food systems and evolutionary nutrition to help people eat and live healthier. His studies have taken him to exotic locales around the world, from Tibet to Papua New Guinea, where he has observed how cultures that consume traditional diets and whole foods have dramatically lower rates of such common chronic diseases as heart disease and diabetes. In his approach to nutrition, Dr. Owen adopts elements of our ancestral dietary patterns using modern day foods, a method that has proven to substantially improve health, vitality and lifespan.

James Darcy, based in Vancouver, has a lifetime of international food experience to draw upon in making his contribution to the recipes in this book. A dedicated food folklorist, his passion is the story about the recipe, the ingredients or the history.

Jean Paré operated a successful catering business from her home in a small prairie town for 18 years before founding Company's Coming in 1981. Since then, she has become a familiar and trusted name in the kitchens of the nation.